The BMA Family Doctor G

High Blood Pressure

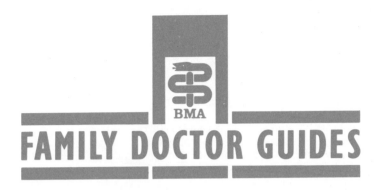

High Blood Pressure

Dr Peter Semple

Series editor: Dr Tony Smith

Dr Semple is a consultant physician at the Medical Research Council Blood Pressure Unit, Western Infirmary, Glasgow.

Published by Equation in association with the British Medical Association.

First published 1989

British Library Cataloguing in Publication Data

Semple, Peter
  High blood pressure.
  1. Man. Blood. Hypertension
  I. Title II. Series
  616.1'32

ISBN 1–85336–053–8

Picture acknowledgements

British Heart Foundation: p. 8; MRC Blood Pressure Unit, Glasgow:
pp. 15, 16; Family Planning Association: p. 31; Westminster
Medical School: p. 42; St Bartholomew's Hospital, Dept of
Medical Illustration: pp. 42, 43; John Rae: p. 75; John Simmons:
p. 76. Diagrams by David Woodroffe; Cartoons by Raymond
Fishwick.

Equation, Wellingborough, Northamptonshire NN8 2RQ, England

Typeset by Columns of Reading
Printed and bound in Great Britain by The Bath Press, Avon

10 9 8 7 6 5 4 3 2 1

Contents

1 Introduction

Discovering that we have high blood pressure usually comes as a complete surprise to most of us. Although the condition is very common (one in 10 adults have high pressures recorded at some time in their lives), it does not usually cause any warning symptoms. Often it only comes to light if your blood pressure is checked as a routine screening measure by your family doctor or if you have to have a medical examination for employment or insurance purposes.

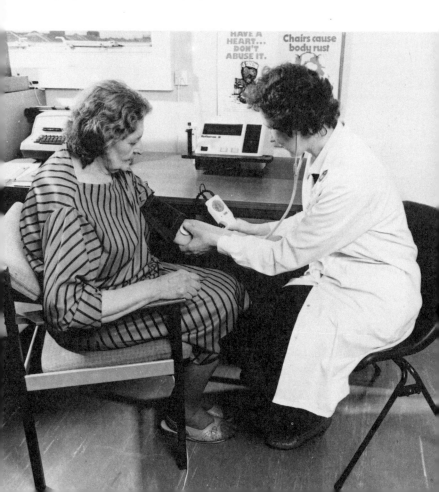

An important health check

If you receive a letter similar to the one below from your family doctor, don't be upset at another and uncalled for sign that you are getting older, look on it as a welcome opportunity to check that all is well. You should always be aware of the possibility of high blood pressure, especially if you are over 40, if other members of your family have it, or if you are overweight.

The Surgery
High Street
Anytown

Date as postmark

Dear Mrs Dunningham

We have just been reviewing the medical records of our patients who have recently had their fortieth birthday. I note that you have not had your blood pressure checked recently. As this would be useful I suggest you make an appointment to see me. The whole procedure won't take very long and I can discuss the benefits of your having this check up when you come.

Yours sincerely,

W.B. O'Brian

pp The Doctors

Benefit of early detection

The main benefit of detecting high blood pressure early is prevention of stroke and heart failure, both major causes of disability and death in this country. It is unfortunate that so many people only discover that they have high blood pressure after they have suffered a stroke or some other complication such as kidney damage has developed.

Treatment is simple and effective

For most people with high blood pressure, treatment is simple and effective and does not affect the quality of their life. Treatment can be tailored to individual needs and any side effects can usually be prevented or overcome. So don't be downcast if you are told you have high blood pressure. Although you may have to take tablets for the forseeable future, be reassured that you have reduced your risk of developing some serious conditions later on.

2 Blood pressure and its measurement

Your heart is a pump that sends bright red, oxygen-rich blood from your lungs through the arteries. These arteries divide into smaller and smaller branches to end in a wide network of tiny, thin-walled blood vessels or capillaries, which are only five millionths of a metre in width and allow only one blood cell through at a time. The blood in the capillaries releases its oxygen into the tissues of the body. Blood that has lost its oxygen becomes blue in colour, and this blue blood is returned to the heart through a system of veins. You can see some of these veins under the skin on the inside of your arms.

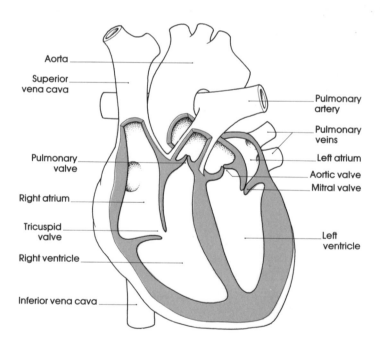

The heart with its main arteries and veins

Arteries under pressure

The pressure in arteries is high but the pressure in capillaries and veins is much lower and it is the pressure in the arteries that pushes the blood around your body. This arterial pressure is maintained by a combination of the pumping action of the heart and a squeezing effect on the blood caused by the tension in the relatively thick and muscular walls of small arteries.

Systolic and diastolic pressures

The pressure inside an artery is greatest while the heart muscle is contracting and this pressure peak is called the *systolic pressure*. Between beats the heart relaxes and the pressure in the arteries falls somewhat. This pressure during relaxation is called the *diastolic pressure*. For a normal young person at rest a typical systolic pressure might be equivalent to 120 millimetres of mercury (mmHg) with the diastolic pressure lower at 80 mmHg. This is written as 120/80 mmHg.

Elasticity

The walls of the large arteries contain a large proportion of elastic tissue. This 'give', or elasticity, gets less with age and some people lose the elastic tissue in their large arteries more rapidly than others. The loss of elasticity results in an increase in the systolic but not in diastolic pressure.

Pressure varies

The pressure in arteries varies considerably throughout the day depending on your alertness, stress, physical and mental activity, and other factors. Blood pressure is usually at its highest in the morning and afternoon and falls in the evening to reach its lowest point in the early hours of the morning and during sleep.

Detecting changes in pressure

All these processes are quite automatic and most of us cannot readily tell whether our blood pressure is high or low. Knowledge of this variation in blood pressure comes from measurements with specialised and expensive equipment that records patients' blood pressure either continuously or at intervals through the day. These measurements are often called 'ambulatory recordings' and are only carried out at a few medical centres.

Symptoms

Less than a tenth of people with high blood pressure have any symptoms and these symptoms only develop if blood pressure is very high. If pressure suddenly falls, too little oxygen reaches the brain and this results in loss of consciousness (a faint in a soldier on parade is a good example of this).

Measuring blood pressure

The first attempt to measure arterial pressure was made in the 18th century when a clergyman called Stephen Hales placed a tube directly in an artery of a horse. This direct method was bad for the horse (and probably very messy) but fortunately medical science has advanced since then and simple, indirect methods of measuring blood pressure have been known of for at least 80 years or more. The method in common use today was discovered by a young Russian surgeon, Nikolai Korotkoff, in the first decade of this century.

Indirect method

The indirect method entails the use of a simple machine called a *sphygmomanometer*. (The first part of the name comes from sphygmos which means 'pulse' in classical Greek.) A cloth cuff or bandage containing an inflatable rubber bag is wrapped around the upper arm with the centre of the bag (or bladder) positioned over the main artery to the forearm (the brachial artery). The bag can be inflated by squeezing the rubber bulb attached to it by a tube. The bulb has a screw cap which can

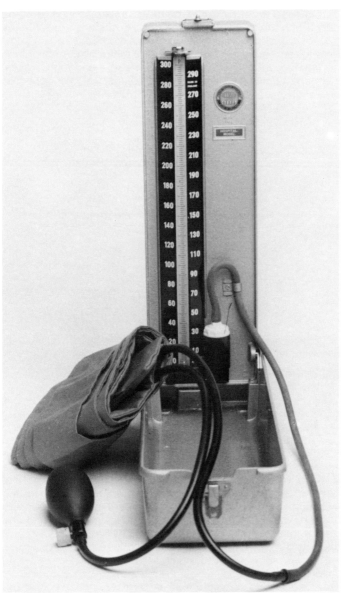

The mercury column sphygmomanometer familiar to most patients

13

be released to let air out of the bag. A second tube from the bag is connected to a pressure gauge, which is usually in the form of a glass tube filled with mercury, marked off with a scale (mmHg) and mounted in a wooden or metal box. Another form of pressure gauge has a dial with a needle and this works on the same principle as the familiar type of barometer called an aneroid.

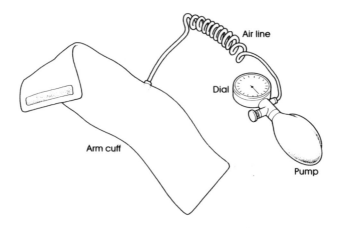

The aneroid meter

With the arm supported at the level of the heart the bag is inflated by squeezing the rubber bulb. As the bag inflates it compresses the arm and puts pressure on the underlying artery. The pressure is increased until the blood flow in the arm is restricted and the pulse beat at the wrist can no longer be felt. Next the bag is allowed to deflate slowly, and by listening over the artery with a stethoscope the doctor can detect the point at which pressure in the cuff is equivalent to the maximum or systolic pressure. Sounds first appear when the pressure in the cuff reaches the systolic pressure and the sounds then continue until a lower point when they disappear and this disappearance coincides with the diastolic pressure.

In some special circumstances such as pregnancy, or in children, the point at which the sounds become muffled is preferred for the measurement of diastolic pressure and this point of muffling is slightly higher than the point of disappearance.

Different sorts of sphygmomanometers

In some measuring devices the sounds are recorded automatically by a microphone that is built into the cuff. These automatic or semi-automatic machines are becoming more popular but there can be problems with accuracy. Measurements may be repeated at will in different positions such as sitting and standing or in different arms. In general, pressure in the two arms is usually the same but there are occasional exceptions to this.

Coin in the slot devices

Various 'coin in the slot' machines that measure blood pressure are often seen in large department stores. They work on the same principle but sometimes are not absolutely accurate. And it is possible that blood pressure could be raised as a result of shopping! If there is any doubt, a measurement should be recorded by someone who is familiar with the technique — a doctor, nurse, or other trained health professional. It is quite easy to learn how to measure blood pressure and most people can become proficient after an hour or two.

Creatures great and small

Cuff size has an important effect on the result of blood pressure measurement in people who are overweight. So if the upper arm is much larger than normal, it is better to use a cuff that contains a larger inflatable bag. In children, the routine cuff size is, of course, smaller. In some children the sounds may be more difficult to hear than in adults, so special techniques using ultrasound may be preferred in infants and very small children. Fortunately, high blood pressure in young children is uncommon except where they have kidney problems and other rare disorders.

DIY blood pressure measurement

A wide variety of machines for measuring your own blood pressure is now on the market and many can be bought for £50 or less. A word of caution is necessary, however. Although some of these devices are accurate, reliable, and simple to use, there are currently no manufacturing standards and accuracy can vary. It is sensible to take medical advice before

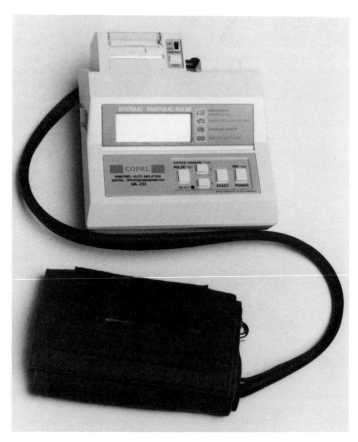

Many automatic or semi-automatic machines are now available

buying one of these machines, or at least to have its accuracy checked against a conventional mercury device. This can conveniently be done by checking the pressure recorded by the machine in one arm against the pressure measured by a doctor or trained person in the other arm with a conventional mercury instrument. It is vital to place the cuff in the correct position on the arm, and this applies particularly to machines that do not depend on a stethoscope. All machines should be checked for accuracy at least once a year.

Is it necessary?

At this point I should emphasise that blood pressure measurements at home are only useful in some people with high pressures. It is definitely not for people with normal pressures. There are better and more accurate and free measurements available. For many people with high blood pressure the condition is treated quite successfully without recourse to home recordings but practice may be changing.

3 Effects of blood pressure

High blood pressure is remarkably common in the developed world and affects up to one in 10 adults at some time in their lives. Probably only about half of these people require treatment with tablets, however. Blood pressure tends to rise as people get older, although this rate of increase is slower in women before the menopause than it is in men. Those of us who are destined to develop high blood pressure often show a steeper rise in pressure with age than normal. This is why it is a good idea to have your blood pressure checked at intervals throughout life — a practice that becomes even more important if a slightly raised value has ever been recorded.

High blood pressure affects up to one in 10 adults at some time in their life.

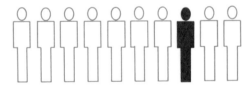

High blood pressure affects on in 10 people

Risk of stroke

A person with high blood pressure has a higher than normal risk of having a stroke caused by the bursting of a small artery deep in the brain. Strokes can also result from a blockage of one of the larger arteries that supply blood to the brain. Many

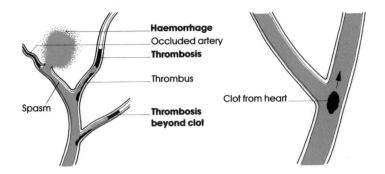

How strokes happen

people will be familiar with the consequences of stroke, which most often results in a paralysis of movement on one side of the body. This paralysis can be temporary or permanent but speech, vision, balance, and feeling may also be affected. Sometimes a stroke is the first sign that blood pressure is high and treatment is then needed to prevent recurrence. Just after a stroke, however, it is often unwise to reduce blood pressure too abruptly. Much depends on the type of stroke and other factors, which vary greatly between people. Strokes sometimes happen to those with normal blood pressure because, apart from high blood pressure, there are other less frequent causes.

Effects on the heart

High blood pressure also puts the heart under some strain, which may cause it to enlarge and function less efficiently. Sometimes this causes no more than undue breathlessness on exercise but in some people breathless attacks occur while they are at rest, and especially in bed at night. Urgent medical attention and treatment is necessary in these circumstances.

Fortunately these heart complications are becoming quite rare and this is largely due to improvements in treatment that have occurred in the past 20 years.

Kidney function

Unchecked high blood pressure can also damage your kidneys, but this does not happen very often and only when blood pressure has been high for a long time without adequate treatment. Treatment with tablets largely prevents this type of kidney damage and can also slow the advance of some diseases that primarily affect the kidneys and are often accompanied by high blood pressure.

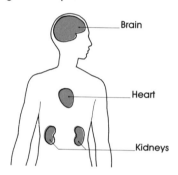

Organs affected by high blood pressure

Blood pressure and kidney function are closely linked and various kidney diseases can cause blood pressure to increase. One kidney disease that can cause high blood pressure at any age is nephritis, or glomerulonephritis. Scarring of the kidneys as a result of urinary infections in childhood is another condition linked with high blood pressure, and occasionally high blood pressure is associated with an inherited condition that causes cysts to develop in both kidneys.

Arterial disease

High blood pressure is one of several factors that can cause fatty deposits or plaques called 'atheroma' to build up on the inside of arteries. This can occur at many sites but the most important arteries that may be affected are the coronary arteries that supply the heart muscle and the arteries that supply the brain and legs.

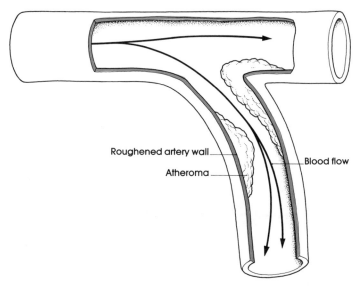

High blood pressure can cause atheroma to develop on the inside of arteries

Angina

Narrowing of a coronary artery can cause chest pain to develop after exercise or emotion and this condition is called angina. During exercise the heart muscle needs more oxygen and therefore more arterial blood. When the demand of the exercising heart muscle exceeds the supply of oxygenated blood, pain develops. This is usually a tight pain felt behind the breast bone but it may travel to the jaws or arms. It is quickly relieved by rest.

Heart attack

Heart attacks are caused by blockage of a coronary artery when a clot of blood forms where there is plaque of atheroma on the inner wall. What probably starts the clot forming is cracking of the plaque on the inner arterial wall. Clots build up and can eventually block the artery, oxygenated blood is unable to get through and this causes death of heart muscle beyond the obstruction. This is the event that is described as a heart attack and it is characterised by a prolonged anginal-type of chest pain that is often severe.

Other factors in heart attack

Angina and heart attacks happen to people who do not have high blood pressure and there are other important causative factors. Most of us are aware that smoking cigarettes greatly increases the risk of heart attack and the risk is also increased if you have high levels of a type of fat called cholesterol in the blood. The amounts of cholesterol in the blood are determined to a large extent by heredity but eating too much dairy produce and animal fat is also a factor.

Are you at risk?

Blood pressure measurements are increasingly used to detect people at high risk of coronary artery disease. Your risk of heart attack can be determined by measurements of your blood pressure and the level of cholesterol in your blood, taken together with cigarette consumption, family medical history, and to a lesser extent, bodyweight. Cigarettes, cholesterol, and overweight are even more important factors if you have close relatives who have had angina or heart attacks before the age of 70 years. Since these risk factors can add together it is important that people with high blood pressure stop smoking cigarettes and reduce their cholesterol levels by eating more fish and vegetables and avoiding too many dairy products and fat. Exercise may help protect against heart disease but this is less well established. Few of these protective measures will lower your blood pressure very much, however, and none are likely to be effective on their own.

Cigarette or cigar smoking remains by far the most important and correctable factor. Pipe smokers may be at slightly lower risk but it is probably better not to smoke at all. The effect of smoking seems to be reversible and the risk of heart attack drops sharply when someone stops.

If a heart attack does occur in someone who is being treated for high blood pressure then less medication may be required for a period of days or weeks until heart function has completely recovered.

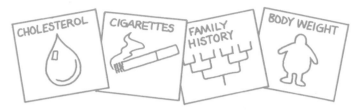

Risk factors for coronary artery disease

Other results of arterial disease

When atheroma affects arteries, such as the carotid arteries which supply the brain, and the artery becomes blocked, an area of the brain is starved of oxygen — you suffer a stroke. Atheroma may also affect the arteries to the legs and when this happens you get cramp-like muscle pain during exercise, which is called claudication. The pain of claudication is intermittent, provoked by exercise, rapidly relieved by rest, and is often felt in the calf of the leg. More severe obstruction causes pain while you are at rest and this is usually felt in the foot.

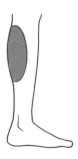

Atheroma may cause a cramp-like pain in the calves during exercise

Symptoms of high blood pressure

In exceptional instances, when blood pressure is very high, symptoms do develop. Symptoms tend to occur most often in children or young adults with kidney disease and in older patients who have developed narrowing of an artery to one kidney as a consequence of the same process of atheroma that can affect the coronary arteries and the arteries that supply the legs. Blurring of vision may then be the first sign of trouble, but of course this symptom can be a sign of another and unrelated eye condition. Breathlessness or a bleeding nose can sometimes be a problem and loss of weight may be a feature. Hospital treatment and tests are indicated in this form of severe high blood pressure and symptoms respond quickly to treatment with tablets. Early detection and treatment of mild and moderate high blood pressure has greatly reduced the incidence of this uncontrolled form of high blood pressure in recent years.

'White coat hypertension'

This term has been coined to describe a phenomenon that is associated with doctors, and hospital doctors in particular. In some people, blood pressure increases when it is measured by a doctor and this tends to be more marked when the measurement is done in a hospital. The effect varies considerably but is a little more evident in young women! Going to hospital is stressful for anyone and this stress is usually greatest at the first visit. Increases of pressure during measurement are apparently less noticeable if the measurer is a nurse or technician and indeed the effect of the doctor on the pressure tends to wear off during a consultation. Doctors are well aware of this potential confounding factor and will rarely decide to treat you after only one measurement of pressure. In most cases several measurements are taken over a period of weeks or months before treatment is started and this applies especially if your blood pressure is only slightly high.

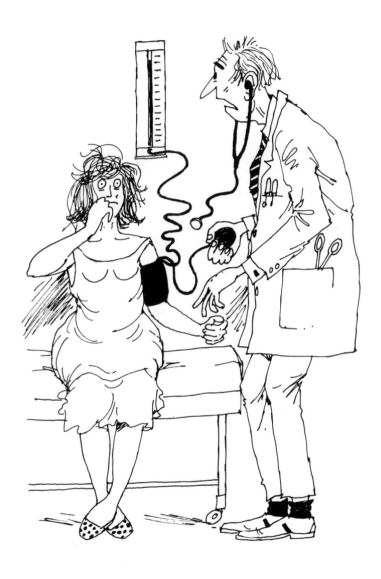

Exaggerating the problem

The importance of 'white coat hypertension' should not be exaggerated and used too readily as an excuse for delaying or deferring treatment in instances where pressures are unequivocally high. Most of our knowledge about the risks of high blood pressure and the benefits of treatment has been gathered in blood pressure clinics in hospitals and with recordings made by doctors!

Low blood pressure

Blood pressure falls in response to bleeding or heart attacks and a sudden fall in blood pressure is responsible for the loss of consciousness in people who faint. With a few rare exceptions there is no condition of chronic low blood pressure comparable to hypertension despite popular belief to the contrary. In general the lower your blood pressure the lower the risk of premature death and the occurrence of stroke, heart attack, and other vascular diseases. There are rare individuals in whom the nerves that automatically maintain the blood pressure on standing fail to function normally with the result that dizziness and faintness occurs, but this is very unusual and is easily distinguished from common and harmless conditions such as simple faints. Faints mostly affect young people and tend to be triggered by prolonged standing in warm environments or sudden emotion and fear and have no great importance for their future health. The tendency to faint gets less as you get older so that sudden loss of consciousness in older people may have other causes and then require more detailed investigation.

Headache and blood pressure

It is a popular misconception that people with *mild* to *moderate* high blood pressure often have headaches. A headache is usually caused by tension or other unrelated conditions such as migraine. *Severe* high blood pressure may be an exception, however, and can provoke a characteristic headache that is often worse on awakening in the morning and tends to be felt in the back of the head. One survey of patients with mild to moderate high blood pressure confirmed that they did not have more headaches than people with normal blood pressure. Headache and high blood pressure only became associated after people knew that their pressures were high. This suggests that headache is then caused by stress related to awareness of the condition — people with high blood pressure expect to have headaches.

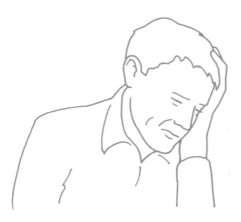

Headache is usually the result of tension or conditions such as migraine

Side effect of treatment

Occasionally, headache is a side effect of drug treatment for high blood pressure. This can occur after taking drugs such as vasodilators (see chapter 7) and some calcium antagonists. In this case the headache is often minor and short lived. If not, it does at least get better quickly when the drug is stopped, and sometimes settles with a reduction in dose.

4 Age, sex, bodyweight, and inheritance

Blood pressure tends to be fairly low in infancy and increases very slightly in childhood with a more noticeable rise during maturation and physical growth in the teenage years. The normal changes and the increase at maturation tend to be more evident in boys than girls and the increase is most prominent in children who become overweight.

Bodyweight

Little is known about the reason for the association of blood pressure with bodyweight but it undoubtedly occurs and the association is maintained in adult life. At this point it is necessary to emphasise that this does not apply to all people with high blood pressure, and indeed not all people who are

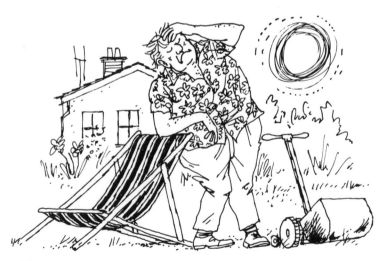

overweight have high blood pressure, but the two do tend to go together. It is natural to suspect that diet is the link but the possibility that inherited factors are important in both has not been excluded. Later in life overweight is a factor in a common type of diabetes that responds to treatment with diet and tablets rather than insulin. The combination of high blood pressure, overweight, and mild diabetes (maturity onset diabetes) is quite common in later years.

Getting the message

The message from these observations is quite clear. It is important to correct overweight by a calorie restricted diet but it is even better to prevent obesity from developing in the first instance. Such a long term change in behaviour is perhaps too much to expect but hopefully could reduce both the incidence of high blood pressure and of so-called maturity onset diabetes. The place of weight reduction diets in the treatment of high blood pressure is discussed in chapter 8.

Inherited factors

After adolescence the rate of rise of blood pressure with age varies considerably. In some people there is very little change in pressure but in others the rise is appreciable. Differences between people are explained both by heredity and by differences in diet, way of life, and other unidentified factors. Factors that are inherited from our parents are probably important in determining whether we have high blood pressure — but we cannot choose our father and mother! The likelihood of developing high blood pressure is about one in three if one of your parents has high blood pressure or has had a stroke under the age of 70 years and this risk increases to perhaps three in five if both parents are affected. Such a positive family history underscores the need for regular blood pressure measurements. If your father and mother live to be over 80 years you are probably unlikely to develop high blood pressure, but there are exceptions. If high blood pressure is the result of kidney disease or some identifiable cause then these family associations are much less important. There are exceptions, however. Some more forms of kidney disease such as polycystic kidneys are inherited and this kidney disease often causes high blood pressure that develops in adult life.

Systolic hypertension

A disproportionate rise in the upper or systolic pressure caused by loss of elasticity in the larger arteries after the age of 60 can lead to a condition that is sometimes called 'systolic hypertension'. This contrasts with the most common kind of high blood pressure where both systolic and diastolic pressures are increased. 'Systolic hypertension' on its own indicates that the blood vessels are older and stiffer, and it does not always mean you need treatment with tablets. People with these stiffer vessels are at slightly more risk of stroke and other arterial diseases such as heart attack but the benefits of drug treatment have not yet been established.

Differences between men and women

Risks of stroke and heart attack are related to the level of blood pressure in both men and women but the risks are distinctly lower in women and this applies particularly to heart attacks. There is probably a true difference between the sexes here, although women do tend to have lower levels of some other heart attack risk factors such as cigarette smoking and it is disturbing that this sex difference may tend to disappear as women increasingly adopt the cigarette smoking habits of men. The benefits of treating women with mild high blood pressure are not as well established as for men and this may be a reason for preferring non-drug measures in women with mildly high pressures but emphasising the need for regular follow up blood pressure measurements.

A word of warning: perhaps a fifth of those with mildly raised blood pressure will develop moderately raised blood pressure over a period of observation of five years and then require drug treatment. All too often the simple precaution of regular checks is neglected.

The contraceptive pill

Many women will have heard of a possible link between raised blood pressure and certain types of contraceptive pills. Contraceptive pills that contain the hormone oestrogen are often called 'combined' pills because they also contain other hormones called progestagens. Oestrogen-containing pills may increase blood pressure in some women, perhaps those with an inherited tendency towards raised blood pressure. For this reason it is routine practice to measure blood pressures before the pill is prescribed and at intervals thereafter. This is done by doctors or nurses at surgeries and family planning clinics and should not be neglected. If your blood pressure does increase then you will be advised to stop taking the combined pill and use alternative contraceptive measures.

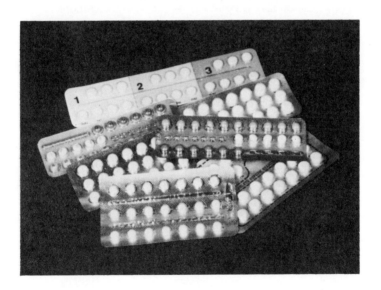

An alternative kind of pill, the mini pill, which contains progestagen only may be suggested. The mini pill probably has little or no effect on blood pressure, although there is a slightly higher failure rate than with combined pills, and irregular menstrual periods may be a problem in some women. Women over 35 years are not usually advised to take the combined or oestrogen-containing contraceptive pill because of a slightly higher risk of thrombosis and high blood pressure.

Hormone replacement treatment

After the menopause, oestrogen hormones may be prescribed to relieve symptoms such as hot flushes and vaginal dryness and are then regarded as a hormone replacement treatment. This treatment replaces the oestrogen hormones that were secreted by the ovaries before the menopause. Hormone replacement therapy may not be suitable for women with high blood pressure, although the low doses that are used for some treatments probably have much less adverse effect on blood pressure than the higher doses that are used in contraceptive pills. Oestrogen hormone creams that counteract vaginal dryness may be safer but it is difficult to determine the amount of oestrogen absorbed by the body. It is difficult to generalise on this subject and you should seek the advice of your own doctor. Blood pressure should be measured at regular intervals in any woman taking hormone replacement treatment.

Women have more contact with doctors

The important question about the safety of drugs that lower blood pressure in women of childbearing years is covered in chapter 9. It is interesting that high blood pressure that is undetected but requires treatment, is less frequent in women than in men. This may be because women have their blood pressure checked more often when they visit the doctor for advice on contraception, or because of pregnancy or gynaecological disorders.

5 Is the cause known?

Although there has been rapid progress in the diagnosis and treatment of high blood pressure, the cause or causes are still not well understood. In most people high blood pressure does not have an easily definable cause but in a minority of perhaps one to five in a hundred a cause can be identified, but specialist investigations are usually necessary. The most common cause that is found is a kidney problem. Many different forms of kidney disease cause high blood pressure but especially those conditions that lead to an impairment of kidney function. Impaired kidney function is easily recognised by simple blood and urine tests but more complex x-ray and other investigations may be called for if these are positive.

Renal artery stenosis

One particular kidney condition deserves a special mention. Narrowing of an artery that supplies the kidney with blood, renal artery stenosis, is an important cause of high blood pressure and a condition that may be helped by surgery or dilatation (stretching the artery). In dilatation a small balloon at the end of a flexible tube is introduced into an artery in the groin and the balloon is positioned across the narrowed part of artery. The balloon is inflated at pressure, thus stretching the area of narrowing and restoring blood flow to the kidney beyond. A cure is not always possible but the high blood pressure usually becomes more amenable to treatment with tablets and kidney function is often improved by successful surgical or dilatation procedures.

Kidney failure

Patients with kidney failure usually require treatment for high blood pressure. High blood pressure is mainly caused by

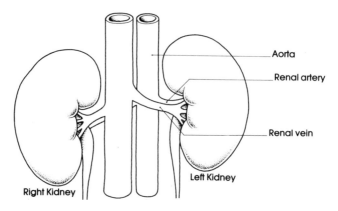

The kidney showing the renal artery

failure of the kidneys to regulate the amount of salt and water in the body. If dialysis treatment becomes necessary, high blood pressure may be controlled by this alone but many patients still need to take tablets too. Blood pressure control tends to be better in the type of dialysis treatment called continuous ambulatory peritoneal dialysis or CAPD for short, than with so-called haemodialysis using a kidney machine.

The adrenal glands are situated above each kidney

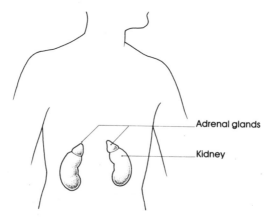

Excess noradrenaline

Other less common but curable forms of high blood pressure are caused by problems affecting the adrenal glands. The adrenal glands are situated just above each kidney and normally have an inner and an outer layer that secrete different hormones into the bloodstream. The inner part of the gland, or medulla, secretes adrenaline, the hormone that is produced in response to fear, anger, and exercise and causes an increase in heart rate. It also produces a related hormone noradrenaline, which constricts arterial muscle and causes a rise in blood pressure. Sometimes a benign tumour or phaeochromocytoma causes a severe rise in blood pressure due to excess noradrenaline in the blood. There may be attacks of sweating, palpitations, and severe headache but the condition is very rare indeed. It is diagnosed by simple blood and urine tests and the enlarged adrenal gland can usually show up on a body scan. High blood pressure caused by too much noradrenaline is initially controlled with tablets but surgery is then curative.

Cushing's syndrome and aldosteronism

Other very rare conditions sometimes result from tumours or overgrowth of the outer layer of the adrenal gland. These secrete either another stress hormone called cortisol or a hormone called aldosterone that causes the kidney to retain salt (or sodium) and lose potassium. Too much cortisol causes a condition known as Cushing's syndrome after the American surgeon who first described it. Cushing's syndrome is very rare and results in rapid weight gain, high blood pressure, and sometimes a form of diabetes. The commonest type is caused by a tiny benign tumour of the pituitary gland at the base of the brain which drives the adrenal gland to secrete cortisol. Surgery is the usual treatment and is generally effective.

Too much aldosterone

Excessive secretion of aldosterone, or aldosteronism, causes high blood pressure with low levels of potassium in the blood. Low potassium can cause muscle weakness and loss of ability to concentrate urine. It is diagnosed by blood tests and surgical removal of the abnormal adrenal gland is often curative.

Cure is not always possible

It must be emphasised that the curable forms of high blood pressure are very rare. It is also fair to mention that some degree of high blood pressure may persist even after successful surgery and still require treatment with tablets. This applies not just to surgery of the adrenal glands but also to dilatation or surgery for renal artery disease. After surgery, however, the requirement for tablets is usually much reduced. The persistent, mild to high pressure may result from structural changes in the small arteries that are caused by long standing high pressure. For 95% or more of people with high blood pressure, however, no simple cause is known. The importance of overweight and inherited factors has already been discussed, but other factors deserve consideration too.

Alcohol

In some instances, high blood pressure seems to be associated with heavy and excessive drinking of alcohol, and blood pressure tends to fall when alcohol intake is curtailed or stopped. This is a factor in about one in ten people and excessive alcohol intake sometimes comes to light after routine blood tests. In general, people with high blood pressure should keep their alcohol consumption down. A safe limit is probably around two small drinks per day with a small drink defined as a single measure of spirits, glass of wine, or half pint of normal strength beer. It is very easy to let your alcohol intake increase slowly and progressively over the years with drinks becoming a routine at lunch and in the evening. Alcohol is now relatively cheap and the alcohol intake of the whole population has increased in recent years. The practice of keeping a drinks diary for a week or two can produce surprising results and sometimes leads to awareness of an incipient drink problem.

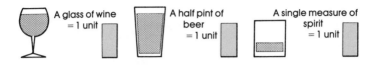

A glass of wine = 1 unit

A half pint of beer = 1 unit

A single measure of spirit = 1 unit

Average British intake (per week)

20 units

Safe limit

Men   21 units per week

Women   14 units per week

Safe drinking limits.

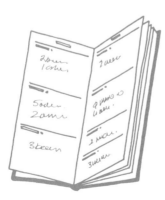

Keep a diary of number of drinks consumed during one week and compare with safe limits above

Stress

There are few people who don't immediately associate high blood pressure with stress but the role of stress as a causative factor in persistent high blood pressure in man is not particularly well established. Stress undoubtedly raises blood pressure in the short term by activating the part of the brain and nervous system that normally controls it automatically. This stress factor has been discussed before in relation to blood pressure measurements in hospital. Stress is difficult to measure and define and this is because events that affect one person do not necessarily stress another. We do not know for sure whether repeated small increases of pressure caused by individual stress will ultimately cause sustained and permanent high blood pressure, but there are clues from experimental work that this may be the case.

Relaxation

Some methods of relaxation and training to cope with stress seem to lower high blood pressures in some people but there is little evidence that outcome is affected or the incidence of stroke reduced by these measures alone. The techniques of relaxation can be learned but relatively few doctors are

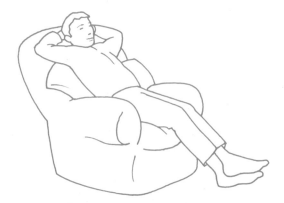

How to Relax

Sit in a comfortable chair or (even better) lie down somewhere comfortable in a quiet, warm room where you will not be interrupted.

If you are sitting, take off your shoes, uncross your legs, and rest your arms on the arms of the chair.

If you are lying down, lie on your back with your arms at your sides. If necessary use a comfortable pillow for your head.

Close your eyes and be aware of your body.

Start to breathe slowly and deeply, expanding your abdomen as your breathe *in*, then raising your rib cage to let more air in, till your lungs are filled right to the top. Hold your breath for a couple of seconds and then breathe *out* slowly, allowing your rib cage and stomach to relax, and empty your lungs completely.

Do not strain, with practise it will become much easier.

Keep this *slow, deep, rhythmic* breathing going throughout your relaxation session.

After five to 10 minutes, when you have your breathing pattern established, start the following sequence *tensing* each part of the body on an *in* breath, holding your breath for 10 seconds while you keep your muscles tense; then *relaxing* and breathing *out* at the same time.

1. Curl your toes hard and press your feet down
2. Press your heels down and bend your feet up
3. Tense your calf muscles
4. Tense your thigh muscles, straightening your knees and making your legs stiff
5. Make your buttocks tight
6. Tense your stomach as if to receive a punch
7. Bend your elbows and tense the muscles of your arms
8. Hunch your shoulders and press your head back into the cushion or pillow
9. Clench your jaws, frown, and screw up your eyes really tight
10. Tense all your muscles together

Remember to breathe deeply, and be aware when you relax of the feeling of physical wellbeing and heaviness spreading through your body.

After you have done the whole sequence (1–10) and still breathing slowly and deeply, imagine a white rose on a black background.

Try to "see" the rose as clearly as possible, concentrating your attention on it for 30 seconds. Do not hold your breath during this time, continue to breathe as you have been doing.

After this, go on to visualise a favourite, peaceful object of your choice in a similar fashion.

Lastly, give yourself the instruction that when you open your eyes you will be perfectly relaxed but alert.

trained in these methods at present. It is probably best to regard relaxation training as an addition to treatment with other methods and it remains essential to monitor the effects of such on blood pressure. Relaxation therapy on its own is unlikely to be effective in people with moderate to severe high blood pressure.

Tranquillisers

Sedative and tranquillising drugs are not now regarded as effective treatments for high blood pressure and their use in this condition is largely discredited. Most tranquillisers can become addictive if they are used for too long and unpleasant symptoms of anxiety and insomnia can then occur when the drugs are stopped.

6 Tests and investigations

A look at the eyes

An assessment of high blood pressure by a doctor often includes an examination of the eyes with an ophthalmoscope and this allows him or her to see the retina. The retina is the light sensitive area behind the lens which translates light and colour into nerve impulses which travel to the brain. Small arteries and veins supply the retina with blood and these small vessels can easily be seen during the examination. In people with long standing raised blood pressure there is thickening of the walls of small arteries and in severe cases tiny vessels burst and cause small areas of bleeding called haemorrhages. In very severe forms of high blood pressure, blurring of vision can be the first symptom. This is distinct from the sudden impairment of vision that sometimes develops as a complication of less severe grades of high blood pressure and then results from blockage or thrombosis of a small artery or vein that supplies

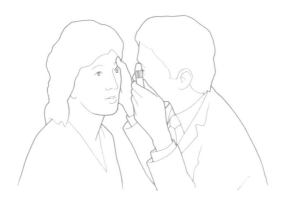

Examining the eye with an opthalmoscope

41

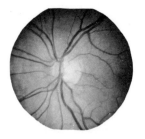

Damage to the retina

the retina. These events are not very common and it is important to recognise that other unrelated eye troubles may occur in patients with high blood pressure, particularly in the older age groups. These problems include clouding of the lens, or cataract, and glaucoma, which is caused by an increase in pressure that is confined to the eye alone. Occasionally high blood pressure only comes to light after a routine eye examination by an optician or doctor.

Urine and blood tests

Mildly raised blood pressures are often treated with little in the way of tests and special investigations but a few simple tests are performed in almost all cases. Detailed investigation at a hospital clinic is less usual. The common tests include urine tests to detect underlying kidney problems and blood tests to measure kidney function directly and these can give clues to the presence of rare and treatable underlying abnormalities of the kidney or adrenal glands.

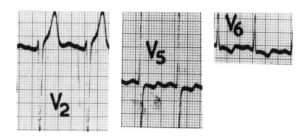

An ECG printout showing raised blood pressure

Electrocardiographs and x-rays

A recording of electrical signals from the heart, or an electrocardiograph (ECG), can show the effects of high blood pressure on the thickness of the heart muscle — an increase in the thickness of heart muscle is a normal response to the increased work of pumping against high pressure. In many instances, high blood pressure is found well before these changes have developed but, even when present, they are readily, if slowly, reversed by treatment. Occasionally, the ECG shows changes suggesting narrowing of the coronary arteries or evidence of previous heart attack. If there are symptoms of angina then an ECG recorded during treadmill or bicycle exercise is often called for. Information about heart size can also be obtained from an ordinary chest x-ray examination. Blood levels of cholesterol may be measured since a raised blood cholesterol value can pinpoint people at increased risk of heart attack and circulatory diseases that affect the legs.

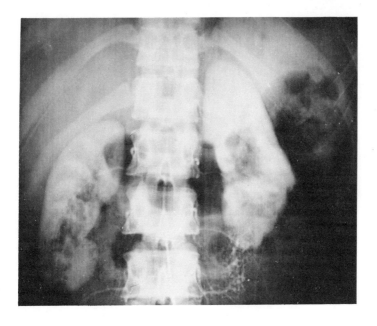

A kidney x-ray showing narrowing of the renal artery

Special x-ray examinations

If the results of blood or urine tests are abnormal or if there are signs from examination or symptoms that suggest kidney or adrenal problems, and particularly if blood pressure is not responding adequately to treatment, then further specialist investigations may be called for. X-ray examinations of the kidneys are performed after injections of a so-called 'contrast' medium into a vein in the arm. Injections carry an extremely small risk of an allergic reaction but it is important that people tell the doctor or radiographer about any previous reactions and about general allergic conditions such as asthma or hayfever. An alternative investigation entails the injection of small and harmless doses of radioactive substances that are concentrated in the kidney and these tests are called renograms or kidney scans. Reactions to such injections seldom, if ever, occur. The pictures obtained are not as detailed as x-rays but if one kidney is damaged or has a reduced blood supply due to the narrowing of the artery then this often shows up on such an examination.

7 Treatment

The main benefit that results from treating high blood pressure is that it prevents stroke. The higher the initial pressure, the greater the benefit from treatment. This is the reason why very high blood pressure requires immediate treatment whereas mildly raised pressures may be assessed by repeated measurements over a period of three to four months or longer before a final decision is reached. If pressure is mildly or variably raised, or both, then observations may continue over a period of years with perhaps some attention to aspects of lifestyle such as diet, alcohol, and salt intake. For all people with moderate and severe hypertension, and for many with mildly raised pressure, continuous treatment with tablets is preferred and treatment of this kind is known to prevent stroke, uncontrolled high blood pressure, heart failure, and kidney damage. Although benefit is related to the initial pressure, the pressure on treatment also affects outcome.

Aims

The aim of treatment is to maintain pressure below a certain target value. This target varies with age and takes account of other factors such as previous occurrence of stroke or heart attack. A gradual reduction in blood pressure is desirable and it is best to avoid sudden large changes in pressure. A slow reduction in pressure allows the circulation and the nerve reflexes that control it to adjust to the new pressure level. This applies particularly to those adaptive responses that maintain blood pressure after changes from lying or sitting to standing up.

Drug treatments

A prime concern of doctors and patients is the matter of drug side effects and quality of life. Although virtually all drugs can cause adverse effects in some people, the incidence of side effects with modern treatment is now quite low and treatments that cause upset can easily be changed. The initial choice of drug depends on factors such as age, blood pressure level, other medical problems, and drug treatments for other conditions. It has been proposed that patients should be given much more information about their prescribed medication and this may come about in the future. In the meantime, let us consider the main types of drug used in the treatment of high blood pressure.

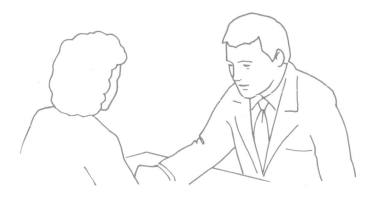

Diuretics

Diuretics or 'water tablets' are commonly used to treat high blood pressure and the type that is most often prescribed is called a thiazide. The popular term 'water tablet' well describes the effect of these drugs on the kidneys — they increase the amount of sodium (salt) and water that is passed in the urine. This loss of sodium from the body causes a slow and progressive fall in blood pressure over a period of several weeks but the overall affect on blood pressure is fairly modest. Thiazide diuretics, and there are many of these drugs, all tend to have the ending '- ide' in their official name and are usually prescribed as a single daily dose which is best taken in the morning. Thiazides are commonly used as a firstline treatment of high blood pressure and have been so used for almost 30 years. They are often given as sole or initial treatment of high blood pressure in older people as they may be a little more effective in them than in younger age groups.

Any problems?

Problems that can occur when you take these drugs are well known and it is unlikely that any major new side effects will be identified in the future. In practical terms, the action of diuretics to increase urine output is usually only noticeable when you start taking the tablets. When you are using them continuously the body content of salt and water is slightly reduced and a new balance between intake and output is then reached. Diuretics may be less successful in lowering your blood pressure if you eat too much salt in your diet. The effect of diuretics on blood pressure is a little greater when you are standing up than in the lying position and occasionally this change of pressure can make you feel lightheaded, especially if you are over 70 years of age. Thiazide diuretics are often given with other types of drugs that affect blood pressure such as beta blockers and vasodilators. These drugs tend to cause the kidney to retain sodium and water and diuretics are useful in preventing this.

Diuretics and potassium

It takes very little diuretic to have an effect on blood pressure in people whose kidneys are working normally, so low doses can be given, which helps to minimise the incidence of side effects. Thiazides all tend to increase the amount of potassium salts lost in the urine and this can sometimes lead to a small fall in the level of potassium in the blood. Usually this causes few problems but too great a potassium loss can cause a feeling of fatigue and muscle weakness and may increase the likelihood of heart beat irregularities. Extra beats can occur in normal people and if this happens you feel as if your heart has missed a beat. Sometimes there is a fluttering sensation in the chest or a feeling of palpitations. Drinks like tea or coffee that contain caffeine and alcohol also encourage this. Extra potassium

tablets are sometimes given to people on thiazide diuretic treatment but it is usually more sensible to increase the amount of potassium in your diet. Vegetables are quite rich in potassium and tomatoes and bananas are a particularly good source.

Sometimes a thiazide is combined with a so-called 'potassium sparing diuretic', which is a different type of diuretic tablet that does not lead to potassium loss in the urine. Drugs of this type are very occasionally used as sole treatment. Potassium sparing drugs such as amiloride are not usually advised if there is impaired kidney function because blood potassium levels may increase unduly. A thiazide is sometimes combined with a newer type of drug called an angiotensin converting enzyme (ACE) inhibitor which also prevents excessive potassium loss in the urine.

Diuretics and gout

Most diuretics increase the likelihood of an attack of gout. Gout happens when crystals of a substance called urate are deposited in a joint between the bones and set up a reaction that causes severe pain and reddening of the skin over the joint. The most common joint affected by gout is the joint at the base of the big toe. Urate normally circulates in the blood as a waste product of body metabolism and spills over into the urine. Diuretics reduce the amount of urate lost in the urine. If kidney function is impaired, the chances of an attack of gout are also somewhat increased. Men tend to be more susceptible to gout than women and the chance of an attack is increased

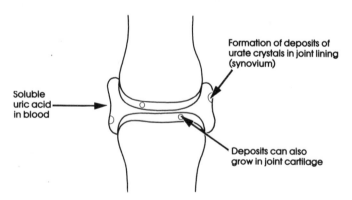

Formation of deposits of urate crystals in joint lining (synovium)

Soluble uric acid in blood

Deposits can also grow in joint cartilage

Deposits of urate crystals in the joint causes gout

by a high alcohol intake and by certain foods such as fish roe, kidney, and liver. Treatment of gout may mean stopping the diuretic and giving a drug that lowers urate levels in the blood. Alcohol intake should also be severely curtailed.

Diuretics and diabetes

Thiazides are probably not suitable for some people with diabetes (the sugar form), a diabetic tendency, or any tendency to high blood sugar levels. This is because blood sugar levels increase somewhat in this group after thiazide treatment.

Sexual function

Diuretic treatment in men occasionally causes impaired sexual function — usually an impaired ability to have or sustain an erection. Fortunately, these difficulties are quite reversible when treatment is stopped. Sexual function in women does not seem to be affected by these drugs.

Loop diuretics

There are also a group of more powerful diuretics that are widely used to treat fluid retention caused by heart failure and other conditions. These drugs are often called 'loop diuretics', a name that comes from their site of action within the kidney. Frusemide is the official name of one of the most commonly used drugs of this type. Frusemide and other loop diuretics are used to treat some people with high blood pressure, but only if their high blood pressure does not easily respond to treatment, if their kidney function is impaired, of if they also have a serious heart condition. Sometimes people with severely impaired kidney function may require very large doses of these loop diuretics to maintain an effect. The thiazide type of diuretics are not very effective if your kidney function is impaired. Frusemide and the loop diuretics tend to produce a brisk increase in urine production for two to three hours only, whereas the thiazide group tend to have a weaker and more prolonged action. If frusemide is prescribed twice daily it is best to take the second dose no later than about 6pm so that the effect is over by bedtime. As with thiazides, loop diuretics can cause loss of potassium in the urine and increase the chances of gout.

Potassium sparing diuretics

Potassium sparing diuretics have been briefly referred to. Spironolactone and amiloride are the official names of two drugs of this type, although spironolactone is now used less often, if at all, for treatment of high blood pressure. Both may be used in larger doses as initial treatment of a rare form of high blood pressure caused by increased secretion of the salt-retaining hormone aldosterone from the adrenal glands (see p. 35). Usually only one gland is abnormal and this can be removed by operation after a period of treatment with potassium sparing diuretic. This condition is most uncommon but may be suspected if you have low levels of blood potassium and these are not caused by diuretics treatment or other medical conditions. Low potassium levels may cause symptoms of muscle weakness and a sensation of pins and needles.

Beta blockers

Drugs of this type are often used as the first treatment of high blood pressure and as part of combined drug treatment with diuretics, vasodilator drugs, and others. Beta blockers were originally introduced and continue to be used for treatment of angina and are also used in some people after a heart attack to prevent a recurrence. The official names tend to end in '- ol'. In general these drugs act by blocking the actions of the stress hormone adrenaline on the heart and blood vessels but they also prevent some of the effects of a part of the nervous system that automatically controls the output of the heart and the tension in the walls of small blood vessels. Some, but not all, reduce the heart rate and slow the pulse beat to around 60 beats per minute or less (normal values are around 70–80 depending on age and physical fitness). The usual increase in the heart rate after exercise is reduced and sometimes you may be aware of the slowed heart beat. Anxiety often causes an increase in heart rate and sometimes makes your hands shake; both these effects are prevented or masked by beta blockers. For this reason there is controversy about their use in competitive sports that require a steady hand such as snooker or rifle shooting.

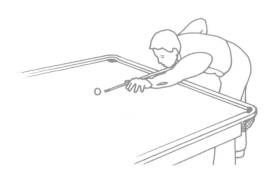

Advantages of beta blockers

Beta blockers are generally effective, tend not to have too drastic an effect on blood pressure, and may be preferred to diuretics in younger patients. They also tend to prevent increases in heart rate which occur in response to treatment with other types of drug such as vasodilators and some of the drugs that are described as calcium antagonists. Beta blockers are usually taken once a day for treatment of high blood pressure but some are taken twice or three times a day.

Problems

The most common problems encountered after treatment with beta blockers are tiredness and lethargy, weak legs, and cold hands (and feet). Many people feel perfectly well, however. Sometimes exercise capacity is reduced and beta blockers are seldom advisable if there is any underlying chest disease, especially asthma or a tendency to wheeze. Beta blockers worsen wheeze in asthma and may cause a wheeze in someone who develops a chest infection.

Undue slowing of the heart beat is occasionally a problem and this can be troublesome in older patients and give rise to tiredness or lightheadedness. People on treatment can check their own pulse rate at the wrist. The aim is to avoid heart rates below about 45 beats per minute. In general, beta blockers have been used successfully throughout the world over the past 20 years and this is a longer experience than many newer drugs such as the ACE inhibitors or calcium antagonists.

Some types of beta blocker may be used for treatment of high blood pressure in pregnancy but individual advice is always needed on this point. A beta blocker should not usually be combined with one particular calcium antagonist drug called verapamil (official name) but may be used quite safely with some other drugs of this type.

Stopping beta blockers

If treatment with a beta blocker is stopped for any reason there is no sudden rebound rise in blood pressure but there may be an increase in awareness of heart beat and sometimes a sensation of palpitations which is present for a day or two after the drug is stopped. This can be a problem in patients with underlying angina and medical advice is needed here.

Calcium antagonists

This name is used to describe the way these drugs work — they reduce the amount of calcium that enters muscle cells in the walls of blood vessels and the heart and reduce the level of muscle tension. The reduced muscle tension in small arteries causes blood pressure to fall.

There are about three different types of drug under this heading and the most common types have names that often end in '- ine'. Two calcium antagonists that have been used increasingly in the past 10 years have the official names nifedipine and verapamil respectively, but there are others. Like beta blockers, calcium antagonists are also used in the treatment of some types of angina.

Side effects

The most frequent side effects after nifedipine treatment are headache, flushing, and ankle swelling. These may also occur to a slightly lesser extent after verapamil, which can also cause constipation. Although nifedipine can be combined with beta blockers, the combination of verapamil and a beta blocker must be used cautiously (if at all) because together they may reduce heart function. Some of the calcium antagonist drugs may have a slight but transient diuretic effect after initial treatment but this is probably not relevant to the effect of these drugs on blood pressure in the long term. The final place of these drugs in treatment of high blood pressure is not yet fully established. Calcium antagonists are also used in combination with other treatments but they may be used as first line treatments in the future.

Angiotensin converting enzyme (ACE) inhibitors

This rather cumbersome name describes a type of drug that has been used in the treatment of high blood pressure for only about 10 years. Drugs of this type are therefore relative newcomers like some of the calcium antagonist drugs. Many drugs of the ACE inhibitor type have an official name that ends in '- il' but other unrelated drugs such as the calcium antagonist verapamil also have this ending. These ACE inhibitors block the effect of a substance that is normally produced by the kidney and acts by constricting small arteries. Drugs of this type are increasingly used to treat high blood pressure but are not yet advised in this country for *first line* treatment of this condition. ACE inhibitors are also used to treat some patients with tiredness and breathlessness caused by heart failure.

Side effects

These drugs are generally well tolerated by most people. There is a small risk, however, that they may cause severe but temporary problems with kidney function in a very small number of people whose high blood pressure is associated with a reduced blood flow to the kidneys due to arterial narrowing. For this reason checks on kidney function are usually done before and during treatment with this type of tablet.

Caution is also necessary because a few people suffer large falls in blood pressure after the start of treatment. This is most likely to occur in those already on powerful diuretic tablets such as frusemide. Frusemide can often be added to ACE inhibitor treatment quite safely, however, and the combination can be useful for some patients. Captopril, which is one of the ACE inhibitors, sometimes causes impairment of taste as a side effect and is also not suitable for people with the rare condition, disseminated lupus. One side effect that has been identified with virtually all ACE inhibitors is a tickly cough, an effect that may not be readily recognised as a drug side effect. The combination of ACE inhibitor with potassium sparing diuretic is not advised because potassium levels in the blood can increase unduly.

Vasodilators

Drugs that dilate arteries directly are often called vasodilators. Some calcium antagonists and ACE inhibitors can also do this but the term is used here to describe a few drugs that are not readily classified under the other headings. Vasodilators tend to be used together with other treatments and one vasodilator that has been used to treat high blood pressure for nearly 40 years is hydralazine. A more powerful vasodilator that is occasionally used to treat high blood pressure when other drugs have been unsuccessful is called minoxidil.

Side effects

All vasodilator drugs tend to cause a slight increase in heart rate. There may be some fluid retention in the tissues causing ankle swelling in some people but these effects may be prevented by combining the vasodilator treatment with beta blockers and diuretics.

Hydralazine given in high doses sometimes causes a rare condition in women, the features of which include widespread joint pains and sometimes skin rash. This disorder can easily be diagnosed by a blood test and is usually reversible.

Minoxidil, which is only used in cases of great difficulty, causes an increase in hair growth and for this reason is seldom if ever used in women. Indeed it has been suggested that minoxidil applied to the head could be a treatment for baldness! Minoxidil is usually only to be used in combination with beta blockers and with powerful loop diuretics which we discussed earlier.

Alpha blockers

These act rather differently from the beta blockers and prevent another action of nerves that automatically maintain the tension in arterial muscle. Drugs of this type are usually combined with other treatments but are occasionally used as initial or sole treatment. Names tend to end in '- in'. The best known alpha blocker has the official name prazosin and is usually given twice or even three times daily.

Side effects

Alpha blocking drugs tend to have a greater effect on blood pressure when you are standing as opposed to sitting or lying and do so by interfering with the action of the nerves that normally adjust the blood pressure to changes in body position. If these changes in blood pressure on standing are too large you may feel lightheaded and this can occasionally be a problem.

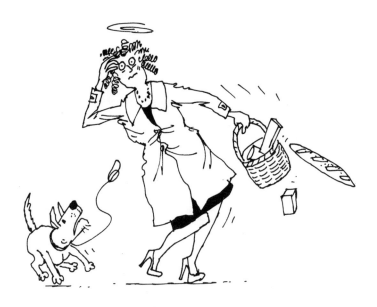

Prazosin sometimes makes people faint after the first dose and if they have been taking diuretics beforehand the probability of this happening is greater. For this reason a first dose is usually taken in bed at night — you are then lying down and won't faint. The manufacturers also produce a special low-dose starter pack of prazosin for the same reason.

Other alpha blockers include the drugs terazosin and indoramin and there is another drug called labetalol that combines the action of a beta blocker with that of an alpha blocker. Alpha blockers including labetalol sometimes cause an unusual tingling feeling in the scalp or under the skin elsewhere.

Centrally acting drugs

The muscle tone in small arteries is controlled by nerves. This happens unconsciously and centrally acting drugs work on the part of the brain that controls the circulation. Centrally acting drugs have been available for many years. One, which has the official name methyldopa, was in use well before the beta blockers. Clonidine, another drug of this type which is used less commonly, is sometimes given in very small doses as preventive treatment for migraine. Centrally acting drugs have mild to moderate effects on high blood pressure and a fairly wide range of doses can be used.

Side effects

The main side effects of these drugs are drowsiness, sedation, and a dry mouth. Centrally acting drugs should be used cautiously if you are taking tranquillisers or drinking alcohol. The effects of the two can add together and result in impairment of attention. Centrally acting drugs may not be the best treatment if you sometimes suffer from depression. Certainly, there is long experience with the drug methyldopa but because it causes drowsiness it is perhaps less used than in previous years.

Clonidine deserves a special mention because a rebound and rapid rise in blood pressure can occur if the drug is stopped abruptly but this is not a risk with the low doses that are used to prevent migraine. Because of the potential for rebound effects on blood pressure, clonidine treatment should not be stopped suddenly without medical advice. A regular supply of this drug should be ensured so that tablets do not run out.

Centrally acting drugs were used as first line treatment at one time and are still useful in some circumstances. There is quite extensive experience of methyldopa treatment for high blood pressure in pregnancy but again individual advice about this is essential.

Drug treatment is effective

This account of drug treatment has not included all the drugs that are used to treat high blood pressure and other types of drug are occasionally prescribed. I have discussed drugs in some detail because they are the only form of treatment that have been shown to be effective in preventing stroke and are therefore the mainstay of treatment in most people with high blood pressure. Other treatments have not been subjected to the same kind of large scale clinical trials that have been done with drugs and none has yet been shown to prevent complications. Many people find it easier to take tablets than to change their lifestyle, especially in the longer term. Do report any side effects of tablets you are taking to your doctor so that treatment can be changed without delay.

Drug treatment in older people

High blood pressure occurs more often as we get older and the overall balance between the benefits and disadvantages of drug treatment may be slightly different in elderly people. For those aged over 65 years, the benefits of treatment are reduced incidence of stroke (as in younger people) but treatment may also reduce the incidence of some forms of heart disease, notably heart failure. The benefits of treatment are generally prevention of disability rather than an increase in life expectancy.

Unwanted effects

The disadvantages of treatment are slightly more evident in older patients and the chances of side effects are a little greater. The mechanisms that normally maintain your blood pressure during changes of posture from sitting or lying to standing, tend to work less well in some old people. A drop in blood pressure on standing may be increased by treatment with some drugs with the result that some people suffer dizziness or even loss of consciousness.

Drug treatments in general are more likely to cause mental confusion in older people, and blood pressure tablets are no exception. Drug treatments are used cautiously in older patients and at lower doses than in the young and it is even more important that schemes of treatment are made as simple as possible and easy to remember. Interactions with tablets used for other conditions are more likely in this age group too since there may be other health problems such as heart conditions and arthritis.

Treatment for high blood pressure is seldom if ever started in people over the age of 80 years, but treatment that was started earlier is often continued, usually at reduced doses. Monitoring the effects of treatment on blood pressure is even more important in this age group and periodic checks on their potassium levels and kidney function are usually required. Older people often keep old pills and medicines with the result that mistakes and muddles occur more readily and the risk of adverse reactions is then increased.

Keeping track of your treatment

There is always the possibility that confusion can occur when drug treatments are started or stopped or doses changed and this tends to happen more often in the early stages of treatment when target blood pressures have not yet been achieved. There is also potential for muddle when both hospital and family doctors are involved in treatment — communications between the two can be delayed. Not infrequently, people just forget the advice that has been given and this is particularly likely if you are anxious during clinic visits. Other treatments may be started by doctors treating other medical conditions and some over the counter medicines occasionally interact with blood pressure tablets.

Carry a card

It is best to carry a card which gives full details of all the drugs you are taking. Cards are widely available at clinics, health centres, and surgeries so do ask for one. Mistakes and drug interactions are less likely to occur if all drugs are recorded in this way. The advantages of such a system are most evident for people with more complicated treatments and with more than one medical problem and it is perhaps a pity that currently there is no standard card available for this purpose.

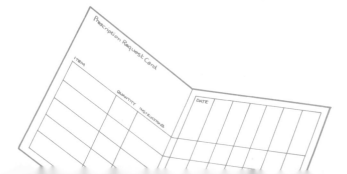

Can other treatments interfere?

It is a common concern that tablets for conditions other than high blood pressure may interfere with blood pressure treatment. Fortunately, interactions of this type are not very common but there are some types of drug that can have such an effect. Most prominent among these are tablets that are commonly used to treat arthritis and other painful conditions affecting the joints and muscles. There is a great number of these drugs and they are known as non-steroidal anti-inflammatory drugs (or NSAIDs for short) and this name distinguishes them from drugs with related effects called steroids.

Effect of NSAIDs

Virtually all of the NSAIDs can interfere with blood pressure treatment and some can increase blood pressure a little in susceptible people who are not on treatment. The effect is fortunately not very marked but can be an important and unidentified factor leading to loss of pressure control which had previously been quite satisfactory. Of course these drugs are essential in many people with painful arthritis, and rheumatoid arthritis in particular, and those who also have high blood pressure may need both forms of treatment. In these circumstances it is often possible to adjust or increase the doses of the blood pressure lowering treatments until the target pressure is achieved, but there can be difficulties.

Pain killers

It should be emphasised that tablets that are available without prescription such as paracetamol, codeine, and aspirin and which are commonly used to relieve headache and minor pain do not seem to interfere with the effects of blood pressure lowering drugs.

Cold cures and appetite suppressants

Some decongestants and 'cold cures' that are used to treat nasal stuffiness and sinusitis can increase blood pressure and should be avoided. Doctors and pharmacists are always willing to give advice if you are in doubt about these treatments. Some appetite suppressants that are only available on prescription also increase blood pressure and may not be entirely safe if your blood pressure is already raised.

Antidepressants

Some drugs used to treat depression may affect the mechanism that normally adjusts your blood pressure when you stand up, with the result that you may feel dizzy. This problem is probably more likely to develop in someone who is already receiving blood pressure treatment. A type of tablet called a monoamine oxidase inhibitor that is very occasionally used to treat depression may interfere with blood pressure treatments but as doctors are well aware of this interaction there is seldom a problem in practice.

Anti-ulcer drugs

A tablet with the official name carbenoxolone which is now used infrequently for ulcer treatment should also not be prescribed if there is high blood pressure without very careful supervision. This drug is related to liquorice which can also increase blood pressure if taken regularly and in relatively large amounts. Those with a passion for liquorice allsorts be warned!

Keep on taking the tablets

The rate of detection of high blood pressure has increased greatly in recent years but it is worrying that so many people don't keep up with long term follow up visits and treatment. This may apply to as many as half of all those who are shown to have high blood pressure. The factors that lead to this 'default' have been hard to identify, although people who are socially isolated and from broken families may be a little more likely to do so. One of the most important, avoidable factors that can lead to default is long waiting times for appointments and long delays in seeing the doctor at the clinic or surgery. It is a regrettable fact that these delays can occur since prompt attention does seem to encourage people to keep appointments and take drug treatments. Continuity of care is another important factor since there is a natural tendency to prefer to see the same doctor or health professional at each consultation.

Keeping up motivation

Duration of treatment is another important variable. Some people find it difficult enough to maintain motivation to complete a simple, short course of antibiotics and it is therefore not surprising that it is difficult to keep up visits to the doctor, blood pressure measurements, and tablet taking, not to mention changes in lifestyle for a period of years and even decades. It may be surprising to some that tablet taking tends to be easier than modification of the way of life since most of us are creatures of habit as far as activity, alcohol, and smoking are concerned. Inconvenience rather than drug side effects is the greatest cause of default from follow up in treatment.

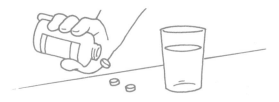

A lengthy process

A single course of tablets is just not sufficient to treat high blood pressure but some people still think that this is enough. Fairly frequent and regular clinic or surgery visits seem to be helpful in the long term and once a month is often about right. It is also helpful to have someone other than the doctor with whom treatment and its difficulties can be discussed. The rate of default from treatment is still too high and there is much room for improvement.

Treatment costs

Under the National Health Service there are charges for each prescription. Most people with high blood pressure have to pay, although some other life-long treatments such as insulin for diabetics or thyroid hormone tablets are free. A leaflet (P11) from social security offices or post offices gives details of those entitled to financial help. At present the main groups that are entitled to free prescriptions are women who are pregnant or have had a baby in the last 12 months, or are aged over 60 years; men over 65 years; and people receiving Income Support or Family Credit.

Season tickets

For those not entitled to free prescriptions it is often cheaper to buy a 'season ticket' or prepayment certificate. These represent a saving if more than five items are needed in four months or 15 items in 12 months.

Application form FP 95 (EC 95 in Scotland) can be obtained from chemist shops, post offices, or local NHS family practitioner committees (health boards in Scotland). These 'tickets' are often the most economical way for people with high blood pressure to pay for treatment. Generally, and to avoid waste of tablets, most doctors prescribe a month's treatment at a time. Longer periods may be more convenient for the patient, but the loss of tablets that results if treatments are changed is correspondingly greater.

Costs to the NHS

The costs of different drugs to the NHS varies greatly. These costs tend to be lower if the official (generic) rather than the brand name is used on the prescription. Tablets that contain more than one drug are called combination preparations and do not have generic names. The range in costs of different treatments for high blood pressure is wide. One year of treatment with a small dose of thiazide diuretic can cost as little as £3 to £4 but a year of treatment with an average dose of ACE inhibitor can cost about £200. Health planners are increasingly interested in the cost effectiveness of different treatments for medical conditions.

A last word on side effects

Virtually all drugs in common use have the potential to cause allergic type of skin rashes. Beta blockers are an example, and may cause rashes and sometimes a feeling of dry eyes. A rash that first develops while you are taking drug treatment should be reported to your doctor in case a drug sensitivity has developed. It may seem surprising but it is possible to develop allergic skin reactions to drugs that have been taken for long periods of time, although problems do tend to occur more often in the early stages of a new treatment.

Many tablets can cause gastrointestinal upsets in a few people and typical problems include nausea, vomiting, pain in the abdomen, or diarrhoea. Symptoms of this kind settle rapidly when the drug is stopped.

Concern for safety

There is always concern about the possible long term effects of treatment that is taken for many years. Drug regulatory authorities are constantly on the lookout for these and fortunately few have been identified so far. Drugs must undergo stringent and prolonged testing before they become available on prescription. In general the longer a tablet has been available and the more people that have taken it then the greater is the chance that it is safe in long term use.

Clinical trials

Drugs are tested in normal volunteers and in patients before they are allowed on the market. People with high blood pressure may occasionally be asked by a doctor to participate in a trial of a new tablet. It is essential that new drugs be tested in this way but you are quite free not to participate and this will not prejudice future treatment. Written consent is usually necessary and people are entitled to a full explanation of all that is involved by the doctor. Even if you agree to take part in the trial you are free to withdraw at any stage.

New drugs are tested very carefully indeed before they are allowed on the market

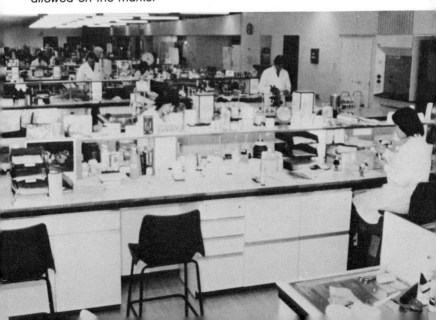

General points about taking drugs

Tablets or capsules may stick at the lower end of the gullet if they are swallowed without an adequate amount of fluid and this can delay absorption into the body. Because some medications irritate the lining of the gullet and may cause heartburn, you should always take your pills with plenty of water or other cold liquid. Some drugs are best taken on an empty stomach, because food can reduce absorption into the bloodstream. An exception is a drug that has caused heartburn, nausea, or pain in the abdomen which may not do so if taken with food or after a meal.

If you are sick

If you develop an illness with vomiting then any tablets that you have taken by mouth may be lost.

This is seldom a problem in the short term except for a drug such as clonidine but medical advice is required if the problem persists beyond 24 hours or so. Illnesses with fever such as flu and gastroenteritis sometimes cause your blood pressure to fall somewhat and your need for blood pressure

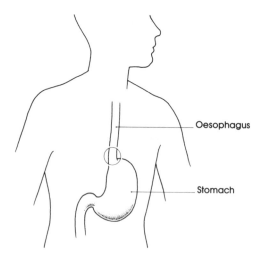

Tablets or capsules may stick at the lower end of the gullet if swallowed without enough liquid

tablets may be less for a period — again medical advice is needed here. Drugs used to treat high blood pressure and other conditions are either eliminated from the body by the kidneys and passed in the urine or destroyed by chemical processes that mostly occur in the liver. Some drugs are processed by both liver and kidney. If kidney function is impaired then the doses of a drug that is normally excreted by this route need to be reduced. With some forms of liver disease dose reductions may be necessary but this is probably less common in patients with high blood pressure. Kidney and liver disease are factors that influence the choice of medication and dose.

8 Self help measures

There is naturally great interest in treatments that lower blood pressure and do not involve drugs, but a word of caution is necessary. Most of these measures have, at best, modest effects on blood pressure and many require changes in lifestyle that may be very difficult to keep up in the long term. If your diastolic blood pressure is consistently above 100 mmHg over a period of time then you will probably need drug treatment. Below this level of diastolic pressure, and especially in women, the benefits of drug treatment are less well established but it seems sensible to try and lower pressures by other methods since even slightly raised blood pressures do carry appreciable risks in the long term. Factors such as drinking too much alcohol and some aspects of overweight, cigarette smoking, and stress have already been mentioned.

Weight reduction

Losing weight if you are too heavy reduces high blood pressure to some extent. The exact effect of weight reduction by calorie restricted diets varies between people and a factor of this effect may be a reduction in salt intake — most calorie restricted diets are rather low in sodium or salt. In general, successful reduction in weight of 5 to 20% can reduce blood pressure by 5 to 20 mmHg. This is equivalent to a weight loss of between 7 and 28 lbs for someone who is 10 st, or between 14 and 112 lbs for someone who is 20 st. Larger reductions tend to be seen if salt intake is also restricted. There is no benefit from weight reduction if your weight is normal and the table gives ideal body weights for people with different types of builds. Very low calorie diets of less than 800 calories a day should only be undertaken with close medical supervision since there are hazards associated with this type of diet and heart problems have occurred in some people.

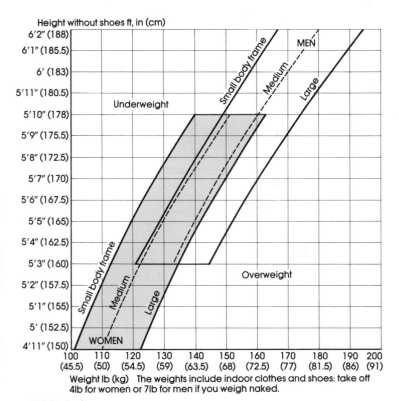

Height without shoes ft, in (cm)

Weight lb (kg)   The weights include indoor clothes and shoes: take off
4lb for women or 7lb for men if you weigh naked.

Weight chart.

Advice on diets

Dietary advice or diet sheets are widely available at health centres, surgeries, and hospital clinics. Information about diets and healthy eating can also be obtained from the health education departments of each health authority and the lists of these publications is given in chapter 12.

There are currently some very low calorie diets marketed under various brand names. These have attracted a considerable amount of publicity and tend to be sold by high pressure sales methods. Most of these diets are expensive — you have to buy special foods which are sold to you as part of a package. Calorie restriction can be done for nothing and motivation can be supplied if necessary by organisations such as Weight Watchers.

Persevere

The rate of initial weight loss over the first four weeks of a diet tends to be greater than in subsequent weeks. Unless this is known it can lead to disappointment or default.

Salt and other minerals

Table salt is sodium chloride. The relationship between sodium in the diet and high blood pressure is a subject of much debate. Interest in the subject has focused on the observation that some small groups scattered throughout the world that have retained a traditional, active, hunter-gatherer way of life have blood pressures that are low and increase very little with age. These groups do not use salt and their diet is very low in sodium but sometimes fairly high in a related mineral, potassium, which is present in most vegetables and fruit. People with these low salt diets such as the Yanomano Indians of the Brazilian rain forests have not acquired an appetite for salt which develops when man or animals encounter salt in early life.

Here in Britain we have an appetite for salt and food with little sodium content tends to taste dull and unappetising to us. A normal intake of sodium in this country is equivalent to about 9 grams of table salt a day but very low sodium diets that are based on rice and fruit and little else can contain as little as 1 gram a day or less. This severe salt restriction is difficult to maintain for very long but does lower blood pressure and indeed this treatment was sometimes used in the late 1940s and early 50s before effective drugs were developed.

Reducing your salt intake

You can, with a considerable amount of effort, reduce your sodium intake to the equivalent of 4 grams of table salt a day or a little less. Cooking is done without salt but it is also necessary to avoid many processed foods which contain salt or sodium glutamate as a preservative. Many canned and preserved foods have quite a high sodium content and there are also considerable amounts in bread, some breakfast cereals, and many dairy products. Fruit and vegetables naturally contain little sodium. If such a restricted sodium diet is achieved then blood pressure can fall about 5 mmHg or a little

The sodium content of some high-sodium foods

Food	Portion size (g)	Sodium (mg)
2 slices of bread	60	160
4 cheese biscuits	30	180
2 tablespoons baked beans	90	430
2″ cube hard cheese	60	365
2 grilled bacon rashers	50	935
1 bowl cornflakes	30	350
1 packet crisps	25	140
1 bowl canned soup	230	1060
Average Chinese take-away	450	600
Hamburger in a bun	100	700
Butter/margarine on 2 slices of bread	20	160
Pickle, 1 tablespoon	30	510

The sodium and salt content of some lower-sodium food portions

Food	Portion size (g)	Sodium (mg)
2 low salt ryvita or matzo	30	6
2 tablespoons low-salt baked beans	90	200
1 small pot soft cheese	60	180
1 bowl puffed wheat	30	1
Unsalted popcorn	25	1
1 bowl home-made soup	230	440
Fish and chips (with no extra salt)	300	330
Salt-free butter on 2 slices of bread	20	2
Apple sauce	30	1

Sources of sodium in the diet

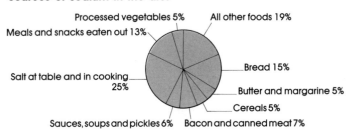

Processed vegetables 5%
All other foods 19%
Meals and snacks eaten out 13%
Salt at table and in cooking 25%
Bread 15%
Butter and margarine 5%
Cereals 5%
Sauces, soups and pickles 6%
Bacon and canned meat 7%

more, but the greatest reductions in pressure tend to occur in people with fairly high blood pressure who are likely to require drug treatment as well.

Is it worthwhile?

Salt restriction may be a worthwhile adjunct to conventional treatment with tablets and may be particularly helpful if you have high blood pressure with impaired kidney function. There are great practical difficulties in maintaining low salt intakes over a long period and relatively few people seem capable of maintaining low salt diets over months and years. Most people with high blood pressure have been treated quite successfully for many years without any modification of salt intake. It is perhaps disappointing that salt reduction has least effect on those with only mildly raised blood pressure since this is the very group where an alternative to drug treatment seems reasonable. There is some evidence that the effects of salt restriction are more noticeable in black people than in white people and there may be slightly more effect in older than in younger patients. Even if you don't adopt a strict low salt diet, however, it seems sensible not to add salt to food at the table and to avoid heavily salted foods such as potato crisps, salted peanuts and salted ham.

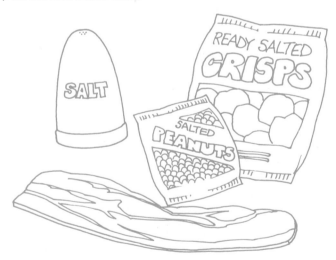

Do not add salt to food and cut down on crisps, salted peanuts and salty bacon

Increasing potassium

Some increase in potassium intake can easily be achieved by eating more fruit and vegetables. Mild salt restriction and an increase in potassium intake are probably desirable for health in general, even if the net effect on blood pressure in the long term is relatively small. Various salt substitutes are now marketed and these tend to be based on potassium rather than sodium salts. Salt substitutes can be used cautiously, although I find that the taste of potassium based salt is not as pleasant as conventional table salt. Some people, however, seem to find the taste quite unpleasant. Potassium based salt substitutes should not be used if you have problems with kidney function or if you are taking some drugs such as potassium conserving diuretics (amiloride and spironolactone are examples) and with ACE inhibitors because excessive increases in the level of blood potassium may occur. Very high levels of potassium cause dangerous irregularities in the heart beat. This is a very rare event, however, and tends only to occur in people with advanced kidney failure.

Calcium

Some people advocate an increase in the element calcium in the diet since there is some evidence that this results in small reductions in pressure. Unfortunately, calcium is mostly present in dairy products such as milk or cheese, many of which tend to have high contents of fat and cholesterol that can lead to undesirable increases in cholesterol levels. At present, I think that the evidence in favour of calcium is not very strong and consider it too early to make any recommendations on the subject.

Tea and coffee

Large amounts of coffee (in particular) and perhaps tea can cause a temporary increase in heart rate and blood pressure but there is little evidence that either substance causes high blood pressure in the long term. If there is any tendency to extra heart beats or palpitations then caffeine in coffee can make this worse. Decaffeinated coffee is best if you have a problem of this type.

Smoking

The adverse effects of cigarette smoking on survival have been emphasised already. Vascular disease of the heart, brain, and legs are all accelerated by smoking. The act of smoking a cigarette causes a temporary increase in heart rate and blood pressure and this is due to the effects of nicotine on the circulation. The increases in pressure are more noticeable in those with high blood pressure. Despite this immediate effect there is remarkably little evidence that cigarette smoking is linked with sustained high blood pressure. Smoking is, however, a cause of atheroma in arteries and this can affect the arteries to the kidney. The resultant arterial narrowing causes a severe form of high blood pressure and this tends to develop in older people with arterial disease elsewhere (see also chapter 3). This is a clear exception to the previous statement that high blood pressure is not in general associated with cigarette smoking. If there has to be priority in the self help measures then stopping smoking should be that priority.

Exercise

Blood pressure increases during exercise but the increases of pressure tend to be a little different depending on the type of exercise. In dynamic exercise such as running or cycling the heart output increases greatly to maintain the supply of blood and oxygen to the exercising muscles. The greater heart output causes an increase in systolic pressure (the pressure during heart contraction) which tends to be greater than the increases in diastolic pressure (the pressure between heart beats). Large rises in blood pressure occur with severe and sudden exercise but the changes of pressure during steady running in someone who is physically fit are fairly modest. After exercise blood pressure falls below starting levels for a period and this can be maintained for up to an hour or more. The rises of blood pressure during dynamic exercise are often modified by blood pressure lowering drugs and indeed there is some evidence that regular exercise can cause a modest fall in blood pressure.

Exercise caution

Regular training with running, cycling, and other dynamic forms of exercise may be good for uncomplicated high blood pressure but great care is needed if the starting level of physical fitness is low and medical advice should be taken in most cases. If you have heart disease such as angina then particular care should be taken. It is often best to follow a formal programme of training and many of these use the pulse rate as a guide to the amount of exercise that should be done at each stage. The rate at which the pulse drops to normal after exercise is an index of physical fitness (see step test overleaf). Severe and prolonged dynamic exercise such as marathon running is probably not advisable if you have high blood pressure. Indeed your capacity for exercise may be reduced somewhat by some drugs used in treatment of high blood pressure such as beta blockers. Exercise is best taken regularly and some degree of fitness can easily be maintained by exercise that is sufficient to cause mild shortness of breath taken two or three times a week. Brisk walking is often sufficient in an older person.

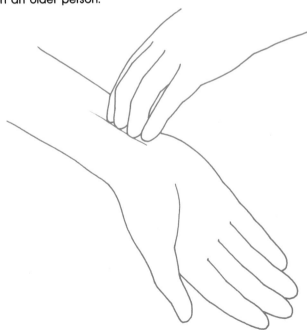

How fit are you?

The step test is designed to assess the efficiency of heart, lungs, and muscles in response to a set amount of exercise. The result gives an indication of almost anyone's general level of fitness. If your pulse rate is in the high 20s you will certainly benefit from a programme of exercise.

Before you try . . .

This exercise separates the very unfit from those of average or just-below-average fitness: Walk steadily up three flights of stairs (each comprising 15 to 20 steps). Do you have to pause for breath, or are you so breathless when you reach the top that you cannot talk normally? If you answer YES, you are very unfit and should consult your doctor before attempting to get fitter.

The step test

Choose a bottom stair — or any fixed platform — about 200mm (8in) high. Step on to it with one foot, bring up the other, and then step back down on to the floor. Repeat the up-and-down process at a rate of 24 times a minute for three minutes. (A test run will help you get the rhythm right.)

WARNING

Do not continue the exercise if you begin to feel unpleasantly out of breath, dizzy, nauseated, or in any way uncomfortable.

Stop after three minutes and wait for exactly one minute. Then check your heartbeat rate by counting your pulse over the next 15 seconds, and this will enable you to read off your fitness rating on the table below.

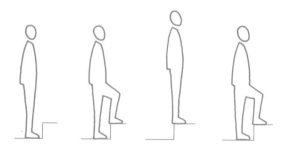

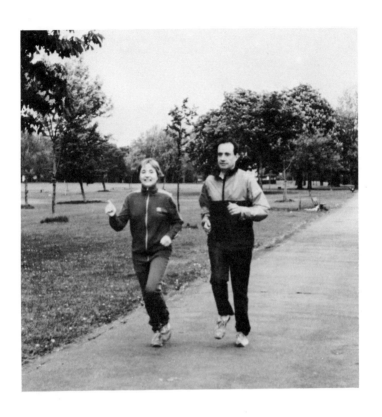

Pulse (heartbeats) counted in 15 seconds				Fitness rating
Men		**Women**		
Under 45 years	Over 45 years	Under 45 years	Over 45 years	
Below 18	Below 19	Below 20	Below 21	Excellent
18 to 20	19 to 21	20 to 22	21 to 23	Good
21 to 25	22 to 26	23 to 28	24 to 29	Average
Above 25	Above 26	Above 28	Above 29	Poor

9 Some practicalities

Having a baby

Women and doctors are rightly concerned about the possible adverse effects of drugs taken in early pregnancy (up to 12 weeks) on development of the baby and much of this concern dates from the thalidomide tragedy in the early 1960s. Some of the tablets that are used to treat high blood pressure are known to be quite safe but others are not yet advised for pregnant women. This is usually not because adverse effects are known to occur but rather because experience of these drugs in early pregnancy is limited. Advice from a doctor is essential here and indeed consultation in advance of the pregnancy is ideal.

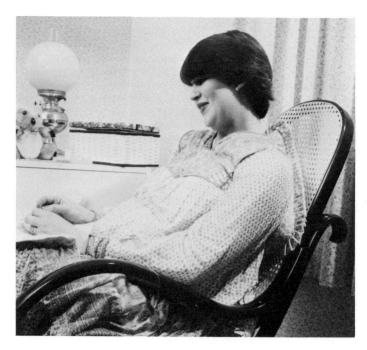

Blood pressure during pregnancy

It is normal for blood pressure to fall a little in early pregnancy with the result that high pressures are seldom found at this stage. In late pregnancy and particularly towards delivery blood pressure may increase in some women and this can occur in women who have never had high blood pressures before. Treatment of this pregnancy associated hypertension is a little different from high blood pressure in other circumstances. Rest may be sufficient to bring the pressure down and this is often ensured by admission to hospital. Fluid retention may lead to swelling of the ankles and protein may leak into the urine from the kidneys and shows up on urine tests. Ankle swelling in late pregnancy, however, is not necessarily a sign of high blood pressure. Urine and blood tests as well as blood pressure measurements are often used to monitor progress and tablets that lower blood pressure may also be given since the baby is completely formed at this stage. If treatments are not completely effective then early induction of labour may be advised and in some severe cases the baby may be delivered by a Caesarean operation.

After delivery blood pressure in the mother falls quite rapidly but it is routine practice to check that this fall is maintained and this is often done at the routine medical examination about six weeks after delivery. High blood pressure may only occur in pregnancy, although there is then a slightly increased risk of high blood pressure in later life in some women.

Driving

High blood pressure has few symptoms and your ability to drive is therefore not affected. Some tablets that are used to treat high blood pressure may cause temporary feelings of lightheadedness, particularly when you first begin to take them or if they are more powerful tablets. If you feel lightheaded avoid driving and go and see your doctor. A few drugs make you less alert and cause tiredness. If your treatment makes you easily tired it is important to break long journeys into manageable stages and to avoid alcohol entirely. The advice about alcohol applies not just to people on treatment for high blood pressure and despite the legal position it is probably sensible not to drink at all before driving any vehicle. Impaired alertness is a little more frequent after the so-called centrally acting drugs such as methyldopa or clonidine. Tranquillisers are not normally used to treat high blood pressure but if you are taking tranquillisers for other reasons you should certainly take no alcohol.

Notifying the authorities

Stroke or heart attack or other relevant disabilities such as epilepsy should be notified to the Driver and Vehicle Licensing Centre (DVLC) in Swansea and it is important to take medical advice before resuming driving after such an event. Licence holders are legally obliged to give this information. Doctors will not normally contact the licensing authority unless you have authorised them to do so and then only in response to a request from one of the medical advisors that are retained by the centre. The licensing centre may suggest and commission a report based on a medical examination. The rules for holders of vocational licences such as heavy goods vehicle (HGV) and public service vehicle (PSV) licences are naturally strict and people with uncontrolled high blood pressure are advised not to apply for such a driving licence. If blood pressure is well controlled by simple medication that is not likely to cause dizziness or other adverse effects and if there are no important abnormalities on an electrocardiographic (ECG) test then a licence may be granted but there is usually a proviso that a medical examination is carried out once a year. Again it is the licence holder that is obliged to report medical problems to the centre, not the doctor.

Insurance

Life insurance companies were early to recognise the relationship between untreated high blood pressure and reduced life expectancy. Because of this some loading of insurance premiums is usual if you have high blood pressure but some companies recognise that treatment works and make allowance for this. It is worth shopping around since the practice varies from company to company. Treatment of high blood pressure must be mentioned in any proposal for life insurance because failure to do so will invalidate the policy. This applies to any form of health insurance that is taken out to travel abroad and to North America in particular where health care can be expensive indeed. It is important to read proposal forms in detail and to consult an independent professional advisor and doctor if in doubt.

Going on holiday

Apart from health insurance to travel abroad, it is necessary to ensure that you take enough tablets to cover the whole period you will be away with a few extra tablets to cover unforeseen delays. Tablets should be clearly labelled with name and strength as well as information about how often you should take them. The availability and cost of drug treatments vary enormously around the world and in some countries drugs are very costly or simply not available. In the countries of the EEC the costs of emergency medical treatment will only be reimbursed by the Department of Health and Social Security if form *E111* has been applied for and granted in advance. The application is made on a form that is obtained at DHSS offices and the period of cover has been recently extended from one to 10 years. Air travel presents no special problems for people with high blood pressure, although once daily medications may need to be rescheduled in due course if there are major time changes. In changing from one schedule to another, it is better to increase rather than decrease the spacing between doses in the transitional phase otherwise excessive falls in blood pressure may occur.

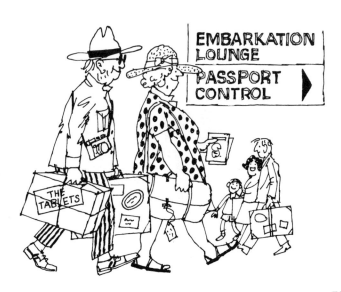

Variations with temperature

Occasionally, in warmer climates, less treatment is required and slight reductions in dosage may become necessary. Such changes are usually fairly minor and it is interesting that there is a small seasonal variation in blood pressure in this country which is probably due to temperature variation. Pressures tend to be a little lower in warmer conditions than in the cold. Saunas sometimes cause large falls of blood pressure in people on blood pressure lowering drugs due to the combined effects of high temperature and fluid loss caused by sweating. The opposite extreme of sudden cold can cause a sudden increase in blood pressure. Plunging all or part of the body into cold water certainly has this effect and similar changes are seen when cold wind strikes the face in winter.

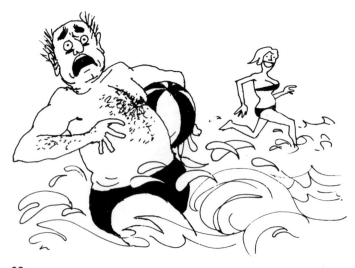

Travellers' tummy and other hazards

If vomiting or diarrhoea develops then medication may be omitted for a short period but should be restarted at the earliest opportunity unless advised otherwise by a doctor. Excessive sun exposure and widespread sunburn are best avoided. There are no particular problems at high altitude (9000 feet or above) over and above the known risks of mountain sickness. This condition tends to affect the young and the fit. It causes headache, drowsiness, and breathlessness at rest and is a particular danger in those who climb too rapidly above 9000 feet. The incidence is increasing as holiday treks to the higher regions of the Himalayas become more popular.

Work

Treatment of high blood pressure usually presents few problems at work and with modern treatment it is seldom necessary to take time off for this reason. In some occupations individual advice is required. A job that involves unprotected exposure to heights such as a scaffolder and steeplejack obviously presents special difficulties because of the risks of lightheadedness after drug treatment. The problems of lorry and bus drivers have already been discussed. The police, fire service, and armed forces usually insist that blood pressures are normal before entry, but often allow individuals who develop high blood pressure to continue to work in some capacity. Special rules apply to pilots and deep sea divers. It is increasingly common practice for employers to insist on pre-employment medical examinations and high blood pressure that is detected or already treated should not prevent people from taking up most occupations. Regrettably, there are occasions when employers look less favourably on applicants with high blood pressure even when the condition is well controlled and the job prevents no special hazards. An independent medical opinion may sometimes be helpful in cases of difficulty. Shift workers may sometimes need to adjust the times at which they take their medication. If a period of night work is likely to exceed two to three weeks then morning dosages should be taken in the evening or vice versa. In the transitional period it is better to increase the interval between tablets rather than decrease it.

Sex

High blood pressure itself rarely affects sexual function, but it is normal for blood pressure to increase during sexual activity. The increases of pressure that occur in people with high blood pressure may be modified by drug treatment. A few blood pressure lowering drugs may adversely affect sexual function, however. Treatment may cause problems with erections in some men and libido may be diminished. These problems are naturally distressing when they occur but are fully reversible when the drug is stopped. Some people may find it difficult to discuss these matters with their doctor but it is important that reticence in the subject does not result in prolongation of distress caused by such side effects. This should not be made an excuse to default from treatment since alternative drugs or non-drug methods are available. The large number of different treatments that give doctors a wide choice and treatment that does not cause sexual difficulty is nearly always available. Sexual problems are perhaps more of a problem in older men than other groups and other factors such as excessive alcohol intake may be relevant in some instances.

Having an operation

People with high blood pressure may need to have surgery for unrelated conditions such as hernia, ulcer, or varicose veins or for more serious conditions such as cancer and heart disease. If there is untreated and uncontrolled high blood pressure then non-emergency operations may be deferred until the pressure is controlled by drug treatment. If surgery needs to be done as an emergency then blood pressure can usually be controlled quite readily by anaesthetics and injected drugs but the risk of heart attack is very slightly increased.

In most cases treatment for high blood pressure is taken up to and sometimes including the day of the operation but the anaesthetist or surgeon will usually advise about this. Treatment is restarted after an interval and this will depend very much on the blood pressure and the ability to absorb medication by mouth. Drugs can be given by injection if necessary. It is essential to take all current medications to hospital with you so that tablets for blood pressure and other conditions can be

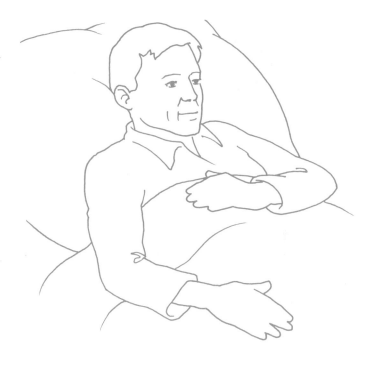

identified and continued during your stay in hospital. It is interesting that high blood pressure often tends to settle somewhat in hospital and this probably reflects the general fall in activity and the process of familiarisation with the hospital surroundings. If blood pressure does settle in hospital then this is not necessarily an indication that higher pressures are not present during the activities of daily life. A large fall of blood pressure during a hospital stay can give a false sense of reassurance.

10 Some people with high blood pressure

Mrs G, aged 50, worked shifts at the local carpet factory. She had three children, the youngest of whom was 14. High blood pressure had been a problem in the later stages of all her pregnancies, and this had meant bed rest in hospital and early delivery of the babies. Although her blood pressure had fallen to normal shortly after having her youngest child, she had not had it checked for many years. A friend at work persuaded Mrs G to attend a well woman clinic which had just been started at the local health centre.

The simple screening procedures at the clinic included a measurement of blood pressure — Mrs G's pressure was high (200/114 mmHg). Other risk factors for heart disease were also assessed at the clinic and a risk score was calculated. An important consideration was the family history. Mrs G had been aged 15 when her mother, who was then 56, had suffered a stroke that eventually led to her death. Although Mrs G was slim and only took a little alcohol, at birthdays and Christmas, she smoked 15 cigarettes a day. Her blood cholesterol value was also slightly high, and this, added to the cigarette smoking and positive family history, pushed Mrs G's risk score up, despite the

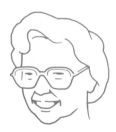

fact that women have a lower risk for heart attack than men. Because of her high blood pressure an electrocardiograph was done and Mrs G had early signs of heart strain, despite the normal heart size that was shown on x-ray.

Because of these heart changes and the fact that her blood pressure measurement was high over a week or two, treatment was started without further delay. At first a small daily dose of a diuretic or "water tablet" was given and Mrs G's pressure then fell slowly over a period of a month to reach around 160/100 mmHg. This was higher than the target pressure of 140/90 mmHg or less, however, and a once-daily dose of beta blocker was then added. Mrs G's target was rapidly achieved and good control has been maintained for five years. In addition her electrocardiograph has returned to normal.

Mrs G and her husband were both persuaded to stop smoking completely. Once this had been achieved it was also possible to lower her high blood cholesterol level by changing her diet. She ate less dairy products and animal fat and more polyunsaturated margarine, fish, chicken, and vegetables.

Treatment for high blood pressure has probably prevented Mrs G from having the same type of stroke or cerebral haemorrhage that disabled her mother. Her risk of heart attack is also greatly reduced since she stopped smoking. Reducing the amount of cholesterol in her diet may also be of benefit in the longer term.

There's nothing wrong with me

Mr S was very cross when an insurance company put up his premiums after the routine medical examination. He was 45, felt in perfect health, didn't smoke cigarettes, and only took a pint or two of beer at weekends. He worked as a salesman for a large company and there had been no comment about blood pressure at a routine company medical five years earlier. Mr S had been anxious about the medical and doctors, surgeries, and white coats always made him uneasy. He was certain that it must have been stress that had caused the high pressure.

Mr S reluctantly consulted his family doctor two weeks after he heard from the insurance company. Although he was much less anxious, his blood pressure was again high at 160/112 mmHg. Every few weeks over the next six months the measurement was repeated, sometimes by the doctor and

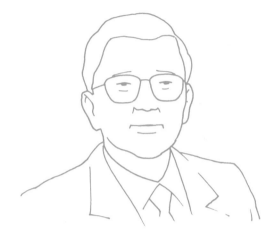

sometimes by the practice nurse. A few simple blood and urine tests were done and his electrocardiograph tracing was quite normal. Although the tests were negative, his blood pressure stayed high, usually over 150/10 mmHg.

Mr S insisted on seeing a consultant at the local hospital's blood pressure clinic. His high blood pressure was confirmed at the clinic but it was decided that some home recordings might be helpful. A clinic machine was supplied for two days and Mr S made recordings at various times in the day. The levels of pressure were lower than at the clinic but still mostly above 140/95 mmHg with some quite high recordings at work in the mornings.

After all the recordings of high pressures over a six month period, Mr S was persuaded that tablets might be needed. He wasn't overweight, didn't drink too much, and kept fairly fit so there wasn't any non-drug treatment that was likely to work. The initial treatment confirmed all his worst fears about drug side effects. He felt terrible – tired, with leaden legs, and was breathless when he hurried up hills. He described it as the "ball and chain syndrome". But the problem was short term. After a week the doctor prescribed an alternative drug and this caused no problems at all. Mr S has now been on this treatment for two years. He is energetic, plays golf regularly, and is able to work as hard as ever. He takes his morning tablet after cleaning his teeth and finds the monthly blood pressure checks when he collects his prescription are a minor inconvenience only. He also uses a blood pressure machine (bought for £40) to measure his own blood pressure and this reassures him that all is well.

Without drug treatment there was a significant risk that Mr S would not survive to retiring age.

But I'm not an alcoholic

Mr P was 50. He had been quite a good rugby player in his day and had even had a trial for Scotland. Since retiring from the game at 33, however, he had lost the habit of taking exercise and had put on quite a bit of weight. Mr P now worked in the oil industry.

High blood pressure was discovered in an unusual way. Mr P was 'electrocuted' when he accidentally cut the cable of his hedge trimmer and was rushed to the accident and emergency department of the local hospital. The shock seemed to have caused no serious injury but his blood pressure was recorded routinely and was found to be 142/96 mmHg. The hospital doctor thought that this raised pressure might be a result of the accident, but a visit to his own doctor for a further measurement was advised. A month after the accident Mr P's pressure was still slightly high at 140/92 mmHg.

There was no evidence of heart enlargement on examination or on x-ray and an electrocardiograph was normal. Routine blood tests showed that Mr P's kidneys were working normally and his urine test was also clear. Blood tests showed that Mr P's cholesterol level was not increased but there were signs of changes often associated with drinking too much alcohol.

Mr P said that he took alcohol every day ... a routine sherry or gin before supper, a whisky before going to bed, and sometimes he and his wife shared a bottle of wine over their meal. Then again there were regular business lunches! Mr P was not an alcoholic but he had to admit that his intake of alcohol had slowly increased over the past few years. The doctor suggested that he keep a drinks diary for a week and the results came as quite a surprise to Mr P. It seemed possible that alcohol was an important factor in Mr P's high blood pressure, particularly since there was no family history of stroke or high blood pressure.

Mr P cut down on alcohol, went on a calorie controlled diet and started to play badminton twice a week. These simple measures have meant that his blood pressure has fallen to around 132/86 mmHg. He is not on drug treatment at the moment, but goes regularly for blood pressure measurements.

A rare emergency — accelerated high blood pressure

High blood pressure does not usually cause symptoms, but occasionally there are exceptions.

Theresa was 15 years old and was taken to an optician by her mother after she complained that she could not see the writing on the blackboard at school. Her eyesight had got worse over a period of two weeks and a shadow had appeared to the right of her field of vision. Theresa had been bothered by headaches, and sports and gym at school made her breathless.

After testing her eyesight the optician looked at each retina (this is the light-sensitive area behind the lens of the eye). He found that there were haemorrhages, or areas where blood had leaked from small blood vessels, on both retinas and suspected that Theresa had severe, high blood pressure.

Theresa was seen by her own doctor on the same day and a very high blood pressure of 240/142 mmHg was recorded. The family doctor referred her to hospital immediately and she was admitted for investigation and treatment.

Theresa's high blood pressure and eye changes were confirmed and a urine test showed that blood and protein had leaked from her kidneys. Blood tests detected a mild problem with kidney function and an electrocardiograph showed evidence of heart strain.

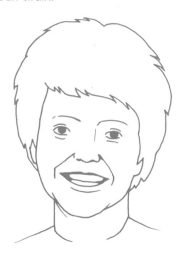

Theresa's high blood pressure needed prompt treatment and a single small dose of a beta blocker caused a progressive fall in the pressure over 24 hours. Eventually a diuretic tablet was added to the beta blocker. Theresa's vision improved over two weeks and eventually returned to normal. The evidence of heart strain slowly disappeared, but slight kidney damage did persist.

The kidney damage was only partly a result of Theresa's very high blood pressure and was a sign that she had an underlying kidney problem. Theresa had a type of kidney scarring that is caused by a reversal of the flow of urine (reflux) from the bladder back up to the kidneys in childhood. This scarring showed up on a special kidney x-ray called an intravenous urograph. The scarring had caused the severe high blood pressure, but fortunately this responded readily to treatment. In the days before drug treatment for high blood pressure was available, 90% of patients like Theresa would have died within one year. Treating the high blood pressure helps to stop or slow the progressive decline in kidney function that often occurs in long-standing kidney disorders.

11 A final comment

I hope that a better understanding of high blood pressure will help to allay some of the anxieties that naturally occur when the condition is first discovered. Effective treatments are now available for a problem that has caused much disability and death in the past but side effects do occasionally occur. This question has been tackled in an open manner out of a conviction that early recognition and discussion of these possible difficulties helps to achieve an early solution and minimise any impairment of quality of life. Adverse effects of drugs tend to be mild and short lived and the wide range of effective treatments means that medication can be tailored to you. Perhaps the most important message of all is that high blood pressure can only be detected and treated if regular measurements are done. Attention to smoking, alcohol, over-weight, salt intake, and exercise can be helpful but medication still remains the mainstay of treatment. The benefits of lowering a high pressure are no longer in doubt.

12 Some useful addresses

- ASH – Action on Smoking and Health, 5/11 Mortimer Street, LONDON W1N 7RH. Tel: 01–637 9843.

  Give-up-pack (send large sae).

- Health Education Departments of Area Health Authorities (Health Boards in Scotland).

  Literature and health education material and information about local classes and activities.

- Health Education Authority (England), 78 New Oxford Street, LONDON WC1A 1AH. Tel: 01–631 0930.

  Publications include: *A Guide to Healthy Eating* and *A Smokers Guide to Giving Up.*

- Scottish Health Education Group (SHEG), Woodburn House, Canaan Lane, EDINBURGH EH10 4SG. Tel: 031–447 8044.

  Publications include: *That's the Limit*, *Beating Heart Disease*, *Food for Thought*, *Eat to your Hearts Content.*

- Welsh Health Prevention Authority, Heron House, 35–43 New Port Road, CARDIFF CF92 1SB. Tel: 0222–471234.

  Publications include: *Exercise. Why Bother?* Runs Heartbeat Wales Programe.

- Coronary Prevention Group, 60 Great Ormond Street, LONDON WC1N 3HR.

  Independent charity (for details of membership and free fact sheets send sae).

  Publications include: *Your Heart* — series of booklets.

- Look After Yourself Project Centre, Church College, Canterbury, KENT CT1 1QU.

  Trains people to run local health activities including pulse-monitoring exercise programmes and relaxation techniques.

Regional co-ordinators appointed (not Scotland). Libraries or adult education centres may have details of local classes.

- British Heart Foundation, 102 Gloucester Place, LONDON W1H 4DH.

  Heart research charity — many local offices.

  Publications include: Small booklets on heart problems, high blood pressure etc.

- Alcoholics Anonymous, General Services Office, 11 Redcliffe Gardens, LONDON SW10 9BQ.   Tel: 01–352 9779.

- Social Security Offices.

  Leaflets including FB28 *Sick and Disabled* can also be obtained from Leaflets Unit, PO Box 21, Stanmore, MIDDLESEX HA7 1AY.

Index